D1285170

An Educator's Manual:

**What educators need to know about students
with brain injury**

Edited by
RONALD C. SAVAGE, ED.D.
GARY F. WOLCOTT, M.ED.

© Copyright by Brain Injury Association, Inc.

No part of this publication may be reproduced, transmitted, transcribed, stored in a retrieval system, or translated into any language in any form by any means without the written permission of the Brain Injury Association, Inc., with the exception of Chapter IV: Families and Educators: Creating Partnerships for Students with Brain Injuries, by Marilyn Lash, M.S.W., who hereby grants reprint permission for educational purposes.

Published by
Brain Injury Association, Inc.
1776 Massachusetts Avenue, NW Suite 100
Washington, D.C. 20036
(202) 296-6443 - Voice
(202) 296-8850 - Facsimile

Library of Congress Cataloging-in -Publication Data

An educator's manual : what educators need to know about students with brain injury / edited by Ronald C. Savage, Gary F. Wolcott.
     p. cm.
includes bibliographical references (p.   ).
ISBN 0-927093-03-0
1. Brain-damaged children--Education--United States. 2. Brain damage. I. Savage, Ronald C. (Ronald Charles) , 1948-
II. Wolcott, Gary F.
LC4596.E38 1995   95-35975
371.91'6'0973--dc20   CIP

Table of Contents

Acknowledgments

The editors express sincere appreciation to the following organizations for their support of this manual

BRAIN INJURY ASSOCIATION, INC.
Washington, DC

ELIZABETH LAUB GRAPHIC DESIGN
Saratoga, NY

WOLCOTT AND ASSOCIATES
Weston, MA

RC SAVAGE AND ASSOCIATES
Saratoga Springs, NY

THE MAY INSTITUTE, INC.
May Center for Education and Neurorehabilitation
Randolph, MA

Appreciation

The editors express their gratitude and appreciation to Rosy McGillan of the Brain Injury Association for her guidance and support on this project.

Dedication

This third edition of An Educator's Manual is dedicated to the children and adolescents who struggle each and every day to meet the challenges facing them. Their courage, their determination, and their desire to continue to move forward serves as an inspiration to all of us—professionals, families, and friends.

The peak of a mountain is only as high as its lowest valley.
Let us not so much lower the peaks
as raise the valleys.

Foreward

According to the Center for Disease Control, brain injury is the single largest cause of death and disability among youth in the United States. The latest report regarding the incidence rate of brain injury among children and young people is staggering. More than a million children sustain a brain injury every year. Over 200,000 children are hospitalized each year with a brain injury. 15,000 require prolonged hospitalization and among those with severe brain injuries, 50% will have major neurological problems.

The causes of brain injury among children are many, but motor vehicle collisions, recreational injuries, falls, child abuse and assault are among the leading causes. Perhaps of greatest importance is the increasing violence against children. The severity of injury in assaults from guns is of special concern. While most injuries are mild, brain injury has a direct bearing on school performance and social adjustment of children. Often mild brain injury goes undetected or is ignored until educational problems appear. The implications for school systems and educators are very significant. As medical and technological research advances, more and more children will survive severe brain trauma. Partnerships between the acute hospital, brain injury, rehabilitation facility and the schools must be enhanced. More and more schools will be called upon to educate by children and youth with severe physical, cognitive and social impairment. For individuals under the age of 22, school systems are the primary providers of long-term education and rehabilitation. To this end, schools and educators must be prepared and able to assist not only children, but also their families, since brain injury impacts the whole family.

The Brain Injury Association (BIA) has entered into a cooperative agreement with the U.S. Office of Special Education and Rehabilitation Services (OSERS) to enhance the cooperation between families, BIA State chapters, schools and state rehabilitation agencies, and to improve services to children and youth with brain injury.

BIA and the members of the Children and Adolescents Task Force are pleased to present the third edition of "An Educator's Manual." The Manual was designed to assist parents, teachers, and administrators in helping students face the challenge of brain injury. This manual outlines the information educators need to help students with brain injury. With up-to-date information, it is a must for all educators and administrators.

BIA is especially grateful to the volunteers who made this new updated version of "An Educator's Manual" possible. A special thank you to Ronald C. Savage, Ed.D., Gary F. Wolcott, M.Ed., and to the members of the BIA Children and Adolescents Task Force.

GEORGE A. ZITNAY, PH.D.
PRESIDENT AND CEO
BRAIN INJURY ASSOCIATION, INC.
NOVEMBER 1995

Contributors

EVE BERGER, M.A.

JEAN L. BLOSSER, ED.D., CCC-SLP

MARTHA R. BRYAN, ED.D

JOAN CARNEY, ED.D.

ANN V. DEATON, PH.D.

ROBERTA DEPOMPEI, PH.D., CCC-SLP/A

MARY-GARRETT BODEL, M.ED, M.S.W.

L. JEANNE FRYER, PH.D.

THERESA KRANKOWSKI, ED.S., C.R.C., C.V.E.

MARILYN LASH, M.S.W.

ELLEN LEHR, PH.D.

SUSAN PEARSON, M.A.

RONALD C. SAVAGE, ED.D.

BETH URBANCZYK, M.S., CCC-SLP

MARTIN D. WEAVER, M.D., ED.M.

MONA WHITMAN, R.N., M.ED.

GARY F. WOLCOTT, M.ED.

MARK YLVISAKER, PH.D.

GEORGE A. ZITNAY, PH.D.

About the Editors

RONALD C. SAVAGE, ED.D.

Dr. Ronald Savage has worked with children, adolescents, and young adults with neurologic disabilities for over 20 years. Presently, Dr. Savage is Director of Behavioral Health Systems at the May Institute, Inc., a nonprofit human-service organization with an international reputation for education and rehabilitation. He is the former Director of Clinical Services for Rehabilitation Services of New York, Inc. and the past Program Director of Hilltop Manor of Niskayuna (a 72-bed specialized brain injury rehabilitation center for children, adolescents, and adults). Dr. Savage has taught at the elementary and secondary school level as a classroom teacher and as a special educator. He is the former Chairperson of the Pediatric Task Force for the Brain Injury Association and serves on numerous professional and advisory boards across the country.

Formerly, Dr. Savage was a tenured Professor of Education at Castleton State College (VT), a clinical Professor of Neurology at the University of Medicine and Denistry of New Jersey, an Associate Professor of Psychology at Rutgers University (NJ), and a director of other brain injury rehabilitation programs and state associations. He presently holds academic appointments at Tufts University, Department of Rehabilitation Medicine and The George Washington University, School of Education.

In 1988, Dr. Savage and Gary Wolcott spearheaded the campaign to include the diagnosis of "traumatic brain injury" in Public Law 101-476: Individuals with Disabilities Education Act. He is presently involved with Emergency Medical Services for Children (EMSC) training programs, the Office of Special Education, and the Professional Advisory Task Force for the National Council on Disability for the United States Congress. In addition, he is helping state education departments write guidelines for students with brain injuries and creating training materials for educators and allied health professionals.

Dr. Savage has presented at more than 200 conferences, training seminars, and grand rounds presentations in the past four years. He has published numerous articles, chapters, manuals and books on children, adolescents and adults with brain injuries and other neurologic disabilities.

GARY F. WOLCOTT, M.ED.

Gary Wolcott began his career working in the mental health field. He received his master's degree in counseling psychology from Northeastern University in 1976. He has served as an administrator and program director of a number of human service agencies. Wolcott developed and directed a rehabilitation program for five years in upstate New York serving persons with mental retardation, developmental disabilities, and brain injuries. This program provided a wide range of community-based services, including early intervention and preschool programs for children, as well as community residential and vocational programs for adults. In 1985, Wolcott became the Director of Education of the Brain Injury Association, facilitating its educational and professional services.

He established Wolcott & Associates, a management and training consultation firm, in 1989 to provide services to organizations working with persons with brain injuries. This work includes staff training, quality improvement, strategic planning, accreditation, and advocacy for persons with neurologic disabilities. In addition, Wolcott has developed programs and materials for parents and educators serving students with brain injuries. He has created training programs and materials for working with students following a brain injury, on school re-integration, and vocational transition following high school.

During 1993-94, Wolcott served as the education and training specialist and a co-investigator on the staff of the Research and Training Center in Rehabilitation and Childhood Trauma in the Department of Physical Medicine & Rehabilitation at Tufts University School of Medicine/New England Medical Center Hospitals. Currently, he is coordinating the development of a neurobehaviroal residential and day program options for persons with severe disabilities due to brain injuries for Goodwill Industries of Northern New England.

Wolcott has the experience of being a family member of two persons who have sustained severe, life altering acquired brain injuries. During the mid-1950's, his cousin recovered from an automobile collision and weeks in a coma. Despite limited medical and rehabilitation care, his cousin achieved successful integration into a job and his community. In 1983, Wolcott's father sustained a brain injury during a medical procedure that left his father severely disabled. The struggle to obtain appropriate and effective services for his father and family provides a unique perspective on Wolcott's understanding of brain injury and its impact on the family.

I   Educational Issues for Students with Brain Injuries

RONALD C. SAVAGE, ED.D.
GARY F. WOLCOTT, M.ED.

Focus:
Incidence and prevalence of brain injury
Pediatric critical care systems
Public Law 101-476 and brain injury
Key educational issues for students

Introduction

It is called head injury, traumatic brain injury, and acquired brain injury. But it all essentially means the same thing— a person has sustained an injury to his/her brain that may change his/her life forever. In fact, the largest killer and disabler of our children is neither AIDS nor cancer, it is brain injuries. When considering the school-age population of people with brain injury, those individuals under age 21 outnumber all other ages combined (BIA, 1991). Yet, children and adolescents with brain injuries have not received the same recognition or services as have adults with brain injuries.

Each year one million children are taken into emergency rooms with "traumatic brain injuries" resulting from motor vehicle collisions, falls, sports, and abuse or with "nontraumatic brain injuries" resulting from anoxic injuries (near drowning, strangulation, choking, etc.), infections (encephalitis, meningitis), tumors, strokes and other vascular accidents, neurotoxic poisonings, and metabolic disorders (insulin shock, liver and kidney disease). It is estimated by the Brain Injury Association that brain injuries to children between birth and 19 years of age annually result in:
■ 7,000 deaths of children
■ 150,000 hospitalizations
■ hospital care costing over $1 billion
■ 30,000 children becoming permanently disabled.

In addition, age is a strong predictor of the cause of brain injury in children:
■ at least 80% of deaths from head trauma in children under two years of age are the result of nonaccidental trauma
■ preschool-age children are the second highest risk group for brain injury
■ children between the ages of 6 and 12 are involved in twice as many pedestrian/motor vehicle accidents as younger children
■ 220/100,000 youths under age 15 will sustain a brain injury each year. Teenagers, 14-19 years old, are most susceptible to sports and auto-occupant accidents
■ 2/3 of the children under age three who are physically abused suffer traumatic brain injuries.

We used to believe that children were wonderfully resilient little beings who could "bounce back" after even severe trauma. Now we know that children are just as vulnerable as adults, only sometimes it takes much longer for the effects of trauma to be seen in a child since children's brains are still developing. Preschoolers with injuries to their frontal lobes often look fine within a few weeks or months. However, as the children get older and their brains mature, that part of the brain previously damaged may not work as well as it should. Thus, when a child's brain is injured it can have long-term devastating effects on the child and his/her family. Too often children who sustain a brain injury early in life may look "well" at that moment in time, but as the child grows older more serious cognitive and behavioral problems may emerge.

Pediatric Emergency/Critical Care Systems

Recently, through a series of Emergency Medical Services for Children (EMSC) demonstration grants, the care of critically ill and injured children has been improved in many states. Prior to this it was not uncommon for children to be treated by medical specialists with little training in pediatrics or for children not to be treated in Level I trauma care centers. A study by EMSC stated in A Report to the Nation (1990) that the majority of infants, children, and adolescents in the United

States who might benefit from pediatric critical care services do not receive them. Presently, a new national movement is establishing sophisticated and designated trauma services to care for children across the country and to develop a system of coordinated services from hospital to home for all children.

Unfortunately, many of these children are not referred to rehabilitation and/or special education services. The National Pediatric Trauma Registry reported that out of 37,000 pediatric head traumas recorded in the registry from 67 trauma centers, less than half of these admissions were discharged to rehabilitation services and only 2% were referred to special education services despite the recognition of noted cognitive, behavioral, and/or motor deficits in many of these children. Recently, a task force of physicians and heath care professionals through Emergency Medical Services for Children (EMSC) began developing discharge guide lines that emergency and trauma care specialists can use to identify appropriate referrals of children between systems of care (e.g., rehabilitation, special education, outpatient services).

In addition, even for those children who are referred for rehabilitation services, few specialized facilities exist that are dedicated to pediatrics. Hence, children often receive services in "watered down" adult programs by adult-trained therapists. Recently, the Commission on the Accreditation of Rehabilitation Facilities (CARF) created program standards for facilities serving children and their families. Also, in 1990, Public Law 101-476: Individuals with Disabilities Education Act (IDEA), added traumatic brain injury as a specific category of students with special needs.

Thus, we now have the beginnings of a national effort to improve the health of children who sustain life-threatening injuries or illnesses. These efforts will focus on developing coordinated medical care services, educating professionals who serve children, collecting data to identify needs, developing continuous quality improvement methodology, creating prevention programs, expanding rehabilitation and community services, and eliminating financial barriers to health care.

Thus, we now have the beginnings of a national effort to improve the health of children who sustain life-threatening injuries or illnesses.

Defining Brain Injury

Ultimately, schools end up being the largest provider of services to children with brain injuries (Savage, 1988; Ylvisaker, 1991). Public Law 101-476 includes "traumatic brain injury" as a category for special education services. New initiatives in states across the country are addressing the training needs of educators to better understand the impact of brain injuries on students. Schools are becoming increasingly involved in working with hospitals and rehabilitation facilities to help students with brain injuries reenter school and plan appropriate educational services. In addition, families and schools recognize the long-term residential, vocational, and social needs of children once the children leave school and home and enter the community.

Historically, in our health care and educational systems, professionals have had a difficult time defining "brain injury" in a way that best identifies those school-age children needing rehabilitation and/or special education services. Physicians, psychologists, educators, and other professionals have often confused themselves with incomplete terms that attempted to describe a person's brain that is not working the way we think it should work, especially after an injury or illness. We have used terms like congenital brain damage, head injury, traumatic brain injury, organic brain damage, minimal brain dysfunction, acquired brain injury, and a host of others to define the "injured brain" without consistency in our definitions (Savage, 1991).

As part of the national Americans with Disabilities Act, in October 1990, IDEA was authorized to include "traumatic brain injury" as a disability category for those students requiring special education services. This disability category attempted to better identify and classify a distinct group of school-age children so that professionals can better plan their educational programs. Traumatic brain injury under this law is defined as follows:

"Traumatic brain injury" means an acquired injury to the brain caused by an external physical force, resulting in total or partial functional disability or psychosocial impairment, or both, that adversely affects a child's educational performance. The term applies to open or closed head injuries resulting in impairments in one or more areas, such as cognition; language; memory; attention; reasoning; abstract thinking; problem-solving; sensory, perceptual and motor abilities; psychosocial behavior; physical functions; information processing; and speech. The term does not apply to brain injuries that are congenital or degenerative, or brain injuries induced by birth trauma. (Individuals with Disabilities Education Act, 1991)

> "Traumatic brain injury" means an acquired injury to the brain caused by an external physical force, resulting in total or partial functional disability or psychosocial impairment, or both, that adversely affects a child's educational performance.

Public Law 101-476 and its reauthorization enables school systems to better identify the needs of students with traumatic brain injury. Schools and teachers across this country have been and are still receiving training about brain injury and the needs of students with brain injury in order to better provide special education services. Many states have set up interdisciplinary teams to develop programs to help students with brain injuries in their ongoing recovery.

Unfortunately, many students with brain injuries acquired from "internal" occurrences do not meet the strict definitional requirements for traumatic brain injury in all states. Students who have had brain infections (e.g., encephalitis, meningitis), strokes and other conditions, anoxic injuries which caused a reduction of oxygen to the brain, brain tumors, neurotoxic poisonings, or metabolic disorders (e.g., insulin shock, liver and kidney disease) are often excluded from the present definition of traumatic brain injury since their injuries were not the result of an "external physical force." Yet, as many educators note, the learning needs of these students are similar to the needs of other students with brain injuries even though their course of recoveries may differ. The educational needs of students with brain injuries generally cluster about three major domains: the cognitive domain, the psychosocial domain, and the sensorimotor (physical) domain.

In medicine, the terms mild, moderate and severe traumatic brain injuries are commonly used to describe the spectrum of head injuries even though no consistent medical definition of these terms exists in present medical literature. Various scales to classify the degree of injury severity caused by head trauma often measure the length of time a person is unconscious, however, many of these scales were normed on adults who sustained brain injuries and not on children. Children often do not experience a loss of consciousness after even a severe blow to the head, nor are their presenting problems as obvious as those similar problems seen in adults (Lehr, 1990). In addition, several major studies of children with traumatic brain injury (Eichelberger et al., 1990; Klonoff et al., 1993; Greenspan and MacKenzie, 1994) have shown that even a so-called "mild" head injury for a child can create significant learning and behavior problems.

Thus, educators are cautioned that the present medical definitions of mild, moderate and severe brain injury may not be the best indicators of outcome or potential for school related problems. Students with mild traumatic brain injuries, for example, may experience problems months or even years later that may be just as disabling as those problems experienced by students with more severe injuries (Savage, 1994).

Education Implications

In educational terms, our brain helps us to think and communicate, have feelings and actions, and move about and interact with the environment. When a student sustains a brain injury, these three major behaviors may become altered, changed, or lost forever. Thus, students may experience problems and need help in three major areas:

Cognitive Needs May Involve:
■ Attention and concentration
■ Thinking and reasoning
■ Communication, language and speech
■ Memory, especially for learning new information
■ Judgment, decision making
■ Planning, organization
■ Ability to adjust to change
■ Perception

Psychosocial Needs May Include:
■ Self-esteem, self-control
■ Awareness of self and others
■ Awareness of social rules and roles
■ Interest and social involvement
■ Sexuality, appearance, grooming
■ Family and peer relationships
■ Age-appropriate behavior

Sensorimotor Needs May Include:
■ Vision and hearing
■ Spatial coordination
■ Speed and coordination of movements
■ Balance and equilibrium
■ Strength and endurance
■ Speech
■ Eye-hand coordination

The return to school can be devastating if the health care facility (hospital or rehabilitation center) and the student's home school do not interact as soon as possible and as frequently as possible

For many students with brain injuries, these needs will be challenging to meet unless we use coordinated, interdisciplinary planning involving all parties: the health care providers, the educators, the family and child, and the community.

Returning to School

The return to school can be devastating if the health care facility (hospital or rehabilitation center) and the student's home school do not interact as soon as possible and as frequently as possible (Carter and Savage, 1988; Ylvisaker et al., 1991; Begali, 1992; Mira et al., 1992; Lash, 1992). The inclusion of traumatic brain injury in our special education laws has helped to improve our understanding of the medical and educational needs of children and adolescents. Hence, as soon as a student is admitted to a health care facility (hospital and/or rehabilitation center), the school reintegration and transition process needs to start. Hospital and/or rehabilitation professionals as part of their policies and procedures need to immediately inform the school that they are presently caring for one of their students and to have the family and/or attending physician formerly request that the school come in and evaluate the child. Under Public Law 101-476 any of three individuals, the parent (or guardian), the child's physician, or one of the student's teachers, can refer a student for an evaluation to determine the need for special education services (i.e., the child's social worker or discharge planner in the hospital cannot).

This evaluation is the important first step in initiating the special education process for identification and classification purposes (i.e., does this student need special education services and how should he/she best be classified). Unfortunately, many students are not referred to the school system for evaluation and are merely discharged back to school with little if any support services in place (Savage and Wolcott, 1994; Blosser and DePompei, 1994). If the attending physician acts promptly and immediately refers the child for a special education evaluation, the school-based special educators or psychologists can then visit the student in the health care facility prior to discharge and decide whether or not this child is going to need special education services and how to best coordinate these services with the hospital or rehabilitation facility. (Savage, 1991; Ylvisaker et al., 1991; Savage and Wolcott, 1994, Blosser and DePompei, 1994).

The IEP is essentially the contract between the student's family and the school system designating the kinds and extent of services the student needs.

Once the school has determined that the student is in need of special education services and has appropriately identified the child or adolescent as a "student with traumatic brain injury," then the school can begin to develop the Individual Education Plan (IEP). The IEP is essentially the contract between the student's family and the school system designating the kinds and extent of services the student needs (Carter and Savage, 1988; Ylvisaker et al., 1991). In the case of those students whose traumatic brain injuries are mild, full-fledged special education programming may not be immediately necessary. Those students may only need to be monitored or have their schedules modified for a period of time to insure that any neurologic sequela has resolved. The school nurse, classroom teachers, and family can then alert the child's physician and/or neuropsychologist, for example, of any persistent problems the student may experience.

For students with more severe injuries, both medical and educational professionals need to recognize that school reintegration is best facilitated by coordinated systems of care, rather than merely passing the child from one system to another. Developing communication protocols between health care facilities, school systems, and families will help eliminate the "cracks" between systems into which many students and their families fall victim. Thus, the initial IEP should be a "joint venture" among the health care facility, the school, and the family. This initial IEP can reflect the cognitive, psychosocial, and neuromotor needs of the student from a functionally-based and holistic approach that will enable the student to become increasingly more involved in his/her school, family, and community as he/she continues to recover. In addition, a student's IEP can even designate the involvement of vocational rehabilitation and community transition services by outside state and local agencies to insure the continuity of services prior to the adolescent graduating from the public school system.

For example, consider the student with a brain injury who is back in school, but is experiencing difficulty remembering historical dates and facts in his/her social studies class. This student may need his/her work area in the classroom restructured to enhance attention and concentration and use specific memory strategies to help store and retrieve information. Therapeutic interventions that worked well in the rehabilitation setting can be carried over into the school setting and such strategies need to be shared with the family to be continued at home. Collaborative planning that starts early in the rehabilitation setting and is extended into school helps merge the health care and school systems with the family into a unified, ongoing program. Again, the IEP is driven by federal mandate and state laws and is the best vehicle we have to negotiate and agree to service delivery models that are in the best interests of the student.

An important component in the IEP process is the duration and timeliness of the educational plan. Many IEPs are written to serve other children with special needs (i.e., students with learning disabilities, behavioral/emotional problems, developmental disabilities, etc.) through an entire school year. However, the needs of students with brain injuries change dramatically as the students continue to recover. Therefore, it is necessary to create IEPs that are not bound by artificial time-barriers. Writing an IEP for a student with a brain injury and not reevaluating the student or the IEP for an entire academic year can have grave consequences. Students and their individual education plans need to be reviewed frequently to coincide with changes in recovery. Children and adolescents with brain injuries, unlike other students with diagnosed developmental or learning disabilities, often continue to make remarkable changes in the first year following the injury. Thus, the IEP needs to incorporate frequent review times to monitor progress or potential problems.

Planning the Academic Program

Health care facilities and school systems that have connected their services have also learned that "school reentry" in not a one time event in the child's life. Returning to school is a series of transitions from the moment the student is injured until they graduate school and beyond, much like a chain has a series of links tying itself together from beginning to end. Unfortunately, many health care facilities may think that once the child is "discharged" their job is completed. Schools may feel that once the child has been identified and classified the student's needs have been met. And parents may feel that once their son or daughter is back home and in school that life will return to normal. Such misconceptions have given many professionals and family members false hopes that all is well and life goes on as before. The reality is that we have a child or an adolescent whose brain is still developing and the impact of the injury to that individual's brain will most likely continue to show up even years after the injury itself (Klonoff et al., 1993; Eslinger et al., 1992; Allison, 1992; Levin et al., 1991; Price et al., 1990). Thus, over time, as school and life become even more challenging for the student, the demands become greater and his/her brain must try to compensate for areas that were previously damaged. For example, a child who seriously damages his/her frontal lobes may function fine in the early years growing up only to experience emotional and behavioral challenges in his/her teenage years. Therefore, when medical and educational professionals speak about "the return to school" it needs to be a carefully coordinated and thoughtful plan that visualizes the needs of the child or adolescent over his/her entire school career and on into adulthood.

For example, in the beginnings of adolescence, young people are confronted with ever increasing cognitive and social demands, more complex academic curricula with as many as 8-10 teachers with whom to work and a host of physiological and psychological changes. Issues of physical maturation and attractiveness, sexuality, self-identity, independence, confidence, and self-worth figure predominantly in the students' evolving lives. Adolescents are "on the go"— driving cars and going out socially. The adolescent with a brain injury may experience great difficulty in any of these areas at a time when he/she also needs to be able to think logically, make adult-like decisions, process vast amounts of information, and solve complex problems. This period of development can leave many adolescents with brain injuries "standing in the dust" of their peers and can create insurmountable feelings regarding the students' losses, inabilities, and hopes for a future outside of school. Such losses can trigger anger, depression, inappropriate behaviors and lead to substance abuse, suicidal thoughts, and academic failure (Lehr and Savage, 1990).

Hence, classrooms, curricula, and teacher responsibilities may need to be reconfigured to meet the student's unique learning needs. Counseling supports may need to be set up to help the student discuss their feelings and learn ways to accommodate socially, and additional family/community services may need to be increased to insure long term success. For example, students may need to "check in" with the special educator each morning to make sure he/she has the right materials, books, etc. for classes that day. Later the student may need to "check out" with the teacher regarding homework, upcoming tests, and any special assignments. The student may need additional speech, physical, and/or occupational therapies integrated into his/her academic schedule through the IEP rather than pulling the student out of school for traditional outpatient services. Classroom teachers may need to modify the academic workload by providing study guides, giving additional time for assignments, or using specific cognitive and behavioral strategies to enable the student to learn more effectively. Such accommodations can enhance the student's recovery and include him/her in school and community activities to the fullest.

As health care centers recognize the need to connect their services with the school, schools also need to connect their services with the outside world.

Often neglected is the issue of post-school experiences (Wolcott and Lash, 1993; Krankowski, 1994). The cooperative planning of where an individual may work, where he/she may live, how he/she will be included in the community needs to begin in the early adolescent years. The involvement of vocational rehabilitation services, independent living centers, and post secondary education experiences are part of the overall series of transitions (Savage, 1987; Wolcott and Lash, 1993). Many young adults with traumatic brain injuries end up living closet lives at home after they have "graduated" from school. As health care centers recognize the need to connect their services with the school, schools also need to connect their services with the outside world. Schools can provide very supportive community-like environments for the student to succeed, but post-school experiences, if not planned for, can become a nightmare. Collaboration with area vocational services, independent living centers, community-based advocacy agencies, and other support systems need to be involved in the student's educational program prior to graduation in order to establish a coordinated transition plan from school to community.

Summary

With the establishment of pediatric critical care systems, new referral guidelines, and the inclusion of brain injury in Public Law 101-476, health care providers, schools, and families have an opportunity to better work together to provide a continuum of services specific to the needs of the child or adolescent with a brain injury. Early referral by the health care providers and the collaborative development of IEPs will enable professionals to blend their services and provide families with a vehicle to insure service delivery.

The chapters in this manual are written by recognized experts in brain injury and are organized to provide readers with a beginning framework to help them better understand the needs of school-age children with traumatic brain injuries. Additional information is available from the Brain Injury Association, Inc. and your state brain injury chapter.

Contributed by Susan Pearson

Melissa

On June 30th, Melissa's mother had just finished classes at the local community college and had picked up Melissa and her five-year-old sister from the babysitter's house. It was about 3:30 p.m. when Melissa climbed onto her bicycle to ride home. She was not wearing a helmet. As she crossed the street, Melissa collided with a car. She was rushed to a local trauma center where the neurosurgeon said she was very close to death. Melissa's injury had caused severe swelling of the brain and as a result, she was put into a barbiturate coma to slow this reaction. As her condition continued to deteriorate, doctors performed a craniotomy which provided additional room to accommodate the brain swelling. The bone was frozen, so it could be replaced several months later. Melissa had been in a coma for a little over two weeks and had sustained damage to the frontal and temporal areas of the brain. Shortly after her surgery, Melissa's condition began to improve and in early August, she was discharged from the acute care hospital and admitted to a rehabilitation center.

Two weeks before her scheduled discharge from the rehabilitation center, staff members felt that Melissa had regained many skills. Her speech production was good and she was independent for feeding and dressing, although she needed occasional assistance with some fine motor activities such as opening milk cartons. Melissa's handwriting also appeared unaffected aside from the fact that she was very slow in completing written work.

Staff members were, however, concerned about Melissa's poor balance. When home on weekend pass, she fell and broke her finger. There was a particular concern about protecting her head, since the protective skull bone had not yet been replaced. Melissa wore a "crani cap" at all times for protection.

Staff members had other concerns as well. Melissa's visual hearing status was questionable; her attention was poor and she was extremely distractible. She also exhibited difficulty with organization and was pre-occupied with toys, food and movies. Melissa frequently confused fact with fantasy, weaving television stories into her own life activities.

Prior to her discharge from the rehabilitation facility, two staffings were held with local education personnel and rehabilitation staff in attendance, in order to share information and to identify what Melissa's needs would be once she returned to school. The second staffing included Melissa's mother.

Prior to Melissa's school re-entry, the local brain injury team (special education staff) spent an afternoon with the students and teachers in the third-, fourth-, fifth- and sixth-grade classes. This time was spent talking about how the brain can be injured and the effects of brain injury on someone's performance and personality. With permission from Melissa's mother, specific information was shared about Melissa's brain injury and how it had affected her. The students and teachers were then encouraged to ask questions and share their concerns. At the end of each session, some time was spent talking about how brain injuries can be prevented.

After Melissa's discharge from the rehabilitation facility, it was determined that homebound instruction would be most appropriate to allow her time to gradually adjust to academic expectations and the demands of a school schedule. After approximately one month, a follow-up evaluation was conducted to determine specific needs for school re-entry. Information gathered during this evaluation, including parent and tutor reports, indicated that Melissa was exhibiting inappropriate social behavior. She was uninhibited in her interactions with strangers (hugging and inappropriate comments) and frequently climbed onto her mother's lap to hug. Her mother also reported inappropriate sexual behavior/activity at home. She was also observed engaging in immature and inappropriate play with toys. In addition to these observations, it was noted Melissa was gaining weight, had a bilateral hearing loss and experienced fatigue after just a few hours. She had also started to engage in ritualistic behaviors such as hand washing, arranging toys and counting things. Motor skills appeared to be within normal limits, as did her speech production.

As a result of these observations, the following suggestions/recommendations were made for Melissa's re-entry to school;
1) full-time aide, at least initially
2) reduced schedule at school
3) special classroom to provide additional assistance with organization
4) no physical education activity until replacement of skull bone; adapted physical education required; supervised travel in the hallway and playground
5) case manager to assist with communication between home and school and to work on social skills
6) may be at risk sexually
7) reduced length of assignments; teach word processing skills to compensate for slow work pace
8) needs a structured routine and time for transitions
9) notebook or calendar to help with memory and organization
10) consider extended year programming

After re-entry occurred, school personnel reported that Melissa was exhibiting aggression toward her teachers and toward other students in the classroom, making it necessary for her to have constant supervision. Aggressive outbursts occurred on three separate occasions;

1) an ice storm required that school be let out early and her regular routine for leaving school was disrupted.
2) classroom location was changed without advance notice
3) teacher was joking with the class and Melissa did not understand the humor; thought peers were laughing at her.

When this information was shared with medical staff at the outpatient facility, there was discussion about the possible effect of phenobarbitol on Melissa's behavior. It was decided that after her bone flap surgery, this medication would be discontinued with close monitoring of her behavior and continued follow up.

In this case, preparing the teachers and peers for behavioral outbursts and inappropriate behavior was important; students were encouraged to ignore and walk away from Melissa rather than react, which was a key factor in keeping her safe. Ongoing communication between the medical and educational professionals also assisted in "trouble shooting" and problem solving in a variety of situations.

Understanding the Brain and Brain Injury From an Educational Perspective

RONALD C. SAVAGE, ED.D.

The brain, our brain, is quite elegantly the supreme organ of learning. All that we do, all that we are, emanates from our brain. Yet, few educators in their undergraduate or graduate work receive detailed information on the brain and how the brain learns or what is happening (or not happening) when the brain does not learn well. Ancient philosophers and scientists did not even recognize the importance of the brain as an entity. Even today in the "Decade of the Brain": we are still exploring our own internal universe to try and gain an understanding of how we learn and who we are. An understanding of the brain is essential if we are to try and gain some knowledge of what happens to the brain after a brain injury. This chapter will highlight our present understanding of the brain from an educational perspective, rather than from a medicinal perspective. After all, the brain is our "learning machine."

The brain is not a hard muscle-like substance, but rather a soft gelatin-like organ that weighs approximately 3 pounds in an adult and about 2 pounds at birth. Brain weight increases more than three times between birth and adulthood. It sits within a rough and bony skull and is bathed in a specialized "cerebral" spinal fluid. The brain is innervated by a sophisticated system of blood vessels which carry blood to and from the heart. There are actually three membranes that cover the brain: the outer dura mater (hard matter) which is like a heavy plastic sheet; the arachnoid (cobweb-like) which bridges the brain's many wrinkles and folds; and the pia mater (tender matter) which molds around every tiny crook and crevice on the brain's surface. It is between the pia mater and the arachnoid that a teacup full of cerebrospinal fluid flows like millions of little streams, bringing nourishment and protection to the nerve tissue.

Internally, the brain has four different reservoirs for storing and circulating the cerebrospinal fluid called ventricles. The ventricles are like tiny lakes within the brain that pool the fluid, help cushion the brain and protect the brain tissue when swelling occurs.

If, for example, the brain is injured by a sudden jolt or bang, it reverberates the blood vessels and delicate nerve tissues to pull apart. To complicate matters the brain rubs against the inside of the ragged and bony skull, causing major bleeding. As with other body parts, the brain bleeds and/or swells with blood and fluid, causing tremendous pressure within the skull which compresses the brain into itself , thereby creating further injury. If you were to trip and sprain your ankle badly, you could either tear muscle, ligaments, or blood vessels. The swelling created by all the bleeding and fluid accumulation would cause more serious problems, which is why we would apply ice or cold compresses to our ankle.

The brain reacts in a similar fashion except our skull is not flexible like the skin on our ankle and cannot handle the swelling. Physicians oftentimes need to relieve this intracranial pressure by inserting specialized monitors into the skull and brain to control the swelling and to surgically operate and remove any accumulation of blood (hematomas). In some cases the bleeds may be so small that the pressure on the brain builds up over time and may go unrecognized until the person starts to exhibit symptoms. The important issue here is that the blow or insult to the brain is only part of the problem. The swelling, bleeding, and contusion (bruises) injures the internal neural network and is often pervasive and not just localized at the site of initial impact. Like a three-pound mold of gelatin connected with billions of microscopic threads, a traumatic impact ripples through the entire brain causing many complications. Situations where there is severe blood loss can cause a lack of oxygen to the brain, called anoxia, which quickly leads to brain injury. Many other non-traumatic brain injuries can cause anoxia. People who experience near drowning, heart attacks, suffocation, smoke inhalation, asthma attacks, sudden infant death syndrome (SIDS), and strangulation suffer anoxia, which kills off brain cells.

The billions and billions of tiny cells making up the nervous system are called neurons. Neurons are the "communicators" and other kinds of noncommunicating glial ("glue") cells support and nourish our neurons. Each neuron has three main parts: cell body, axon (a long, slim "wire" that transmits signals from one cell body to another via junctions known as synapses), and dendrites (networks of short "wires" that branch out from an axon and synapse with the ends of axons from other neurons). The neurons receive and transmit information in a relay where electrical impulses flow through those nerve-cell pathways, the axons and dendrites. Neurochemical transmitters leap the synaptic gaps between each neuron's axon and the other neurons with which an axon makes contact. Each neuron is its own miniature information center which decides to fire or not fire off an electrical impulse, depending on the thousand or so signals it is receiving at every moment. After a child sustains a brain injury, many of these pathways may be torn apart or stretched to a point when information processing is no longer possible. The study of nerve regeneration, repair, and creating new neuronal growth will keep many researchers busy for years to come.

Brain Geography

To better understand how our brain helps us to think, move, and act we need to study some basic neuroanatomy — a geography lesson on the brain so to speak. In order to better visualize how the brain looks geographically, take a golf ball in your hand and close your fist around it. Your arm resembles your spinal cord, which receives information from our skin and muscles and relays this information upward and, of course, relays information down and out from our brain. Your wrist is your brainstem, a small but important extension of your spinal cord. It is like the "point person" for all incoming and outgoing information and basic life functions. The golf ball you are holding represents your limbic system, a rim of cortical structures which encircle the top of the brain stem and are involved in our emotions and basic elemental feelings. Sitting atop and enveloping the limbic system, like our hands around the golf ball, is our cerebral cortex divided into two hemispheres which are dedicated to our highest levels of thinking, moving, and acting. Lastly, situated in the lower back of our brain is our cerebellum which coordinates, modulates, and stores all our body movement. This interconnecting system of neural structures makes up our brain and who we are and are becoming. To understand this wondrous geography will better help us understand what happens when the brain is injured.

The Brain Stem

A more detailed look at our central nervous system reveals a major trunk, the brainstem, which evolves from the spinal cord. Our brainstem is made up of three integral areas called the medulla, the pons, the midbrain, and the diencephalon. Our brainstem also contains many of the centers for our senses: hearing, touch, taste, and balance (except sight and smell). It is in this array of brain structures in our brainstem that a collection of nerve fibers and nuclei called the reticular activating system modulates our arousal, alertness, concentration and basic biological rhythms. If you find yourself getting sleepy or having trouble attending to the information in this chapter, you need to "turn up" your RAS. It is much like the dimmer switch on a light that we can turn up to make the lighter brighter, or turn down to make it darker. After a brain injury many individuals lose con-

Each neuron is its own miniature information center which decides to fire or not fire off an electrical impulse, depending on the thousand or so signals it is receiving at every moment.

sciousness, which can result in coma. Because of the severity of the injury or the brain swelling, the person's dimmer switch may be turned down, leaving the individual unable to respond to even simple commands and leaving that person unaware of his/her surroundings. Unfortunately, the RAS can be depressed to a point where life as we know it ceases to exist.

The first "unit" in the lower part of our brain stem is made up of the medulla and the pons which are involved in many of our basic living functions. The first area is called the medulla, which is about an inch of brain tissue that is vital to life and death, as is the rest of the brainstem. The medulla controls many of our basic metabolic responses: swallowing; vomiting; breathing; respiration and heart rates; and blood pressure. This is where the polio virus struck and why children had to be placed in the "iron lung" machines of the 1950s, which assisted with functions the children's medullas could no longer perform. When the medulla is injured, as with any area of our brainstem, life is immediately threatened.

Just above our medulla is the pons, a bridge or broad band of nerve fibers that connect the cerebral cortex and the cerebellum. This bridge of nerve fibers enables the "thinking" part of the brain (cortex) to work with the "movement" (cerebellum) part of our brain. Disruption to the pons can result in the complete loss of our abilities, leaving us partially or totally paralyzed. Injury to the medulla and/or pons can result in serious metabolic disturbances. Sometimes the upper regions of the brain can sustain catastrophic injury resulting in "brain death", but the person still breathes and his/her heart still beats, even without life supporting equipment. In this situation the person is said to be in a prolonged coma or "persistent vegetative state." Unfortunately, this is where the slang term "vegetable" has been used to describe individuals in long-term coma and this erroneously describes the circumstances.

The second "unit" in the upper part of our brainstem contains the midbrain and the diencephalon and is responsible for alertness and arousal. Interestingly, the smallest part of our brainstem is the midbrain, yet, as small as the midbrain is, elementary forms of seeing and hearing are possible. Only centimeters above the midbrain is the diencephalon (comprised of the thalamus, hypothalamus, and other structures). This is a master relay center for forwarding information, sensations, and movement. The hypothalamus, in particular, is the control center for eating, drinking, sexual rhythms, endocrine levels, and temperature regulation. It is also involved in many of our complex responses like anger, fatigue, memory, and calmness, and serves as the "conductor" of our emotional orchestra. The thalamus sits on the very top of the brain stem just beneath the cortex. It acts as a major relay station for incoming and outgoing sensory information. Each of our senses, with the exception of smell, relays its impulses through the thalamus.

Individuals who sustain injury to this part the brain can experience severe attention and concentration problems; difficulty with memory storage and retrieval; weakened mental stamina; decreased sensory information; difficulty in reacting to stress; and disorders in eating/drinking, sleeping, and sexual functioning. Since the hypothalamus is the major brain region which manages the release of body hormones, people with brain injury may end up with many complex problems. The brain is also the largest "chemical" factory in the body. Disruption to our hormonal, endocrine, and/or neurochemical systems can be just as devastating as injury to the neural network.

Sometimes the upper regions of the brain can sustain catastrophic injury resulting in "brain death," but the person still breathes and his/her heart still beats, even without life supporting equipment.

The Limbic System

Situated above, around, and interconnected with the diencephalon is our limbic system, an area of the brain which is likened to the golf ball you are holding in your hand. Many "neuro" professionals (neurosurgeons, neurologists, neuropsychologists, neuroeducators, etc.) argue about which particular areas of the brain best fit into certain systems. Is the diencephalon with its thalamus and hypothalamus part of the limbic system or the upper brain stem? Arguments like these are moot if one believes that the brain is a highly interconnected and complex system that integrates many units into a beehive of internal and external responses and actions. Thus, even the golf ball you hold in your hand is only a gross representation of the limbic system and its connectiveness to the other regions of our brains. While chopping up the brain geographically may help us better appreciate various components and systems, it is only for convenience that we do this.

No single part of the brain can ever be discussed without connecting it to the whole. Just to talk about "attention" involves the brainstem, limbic system, and cortex.

As we take a more detailed look at the limbic system we find increasing complexity and connectiveness with other parts of our brains, especially the cerebral cortex. Some brain researchers have referred to the "middle" part of the brain as the mammalian brain, the evolutionary, animal-like part of the brain that houses our basic elemental drives, emotions, and survival instincts. The two major structures usually associated with the limbic system include the hippocampus and the amygdala. Injury or damage to any of these structures can leave long-term and devastating problems for people with brain injury. The hippocampus is a paired-organ, one on each side of the brain sitting within the temporal lobes. The hippocampus is most commonly associated with memory functioning and is particularly susceptible to loss of oxygen. Injury to the hippocampus causes individuals who sustain brain injury to have a great deal of difficulty with short-term memory, turning short-term memories into long-term memories, and organizing and retrieving previously stored memories. The hippocampus is like the pole in your closet on which you hang your clothes. If the pole was pulled out your clothes would fall into a heap. Your entire system, like the hanging clothes, in certain areas would be completely disrupted. As you go to store new clothes, there is no pole (organizational structure) to efficiently help you. Thus, your clothes end up in a mess on the floor, which makes it difficult to find anything.

Close to the hippocampus is your amygdala, a "fight-flight" structure that seems to be more closely tied with emotional memories and reactions. There is speculation that when a perception reaches the cerebral cortex, it will be stored within the amygdala if it arouses emotions. Our hidden "fears" of snakes, spiders, and creatures of the night may cause us to run or stand our ground depending on the emotional response from the amygdala. Interestingly, both the hippocampus and amygdala are directly tied with our olfactory fibers, which is why many people in the early stages of recovery benefit from smell stimulation — their mother's perfume, familiar clothes, favorite food odors. While all of our sensations — sight, sound, taste, touch — evoke memories, both smell and taste seem to be the most powerful stimulants for recollection.

Injury or disruption to the limbic system can produce a series of complex problems involving our basic emotional responses to the world and ourselves and how we perceive and "feel." Our actions, so often guided by our emotions, can become uncontrollable. We can become locked into over- or under-reacting to even the simplest of situations. One minute everything is all right, the next the

The hippocampus is like the pole in your closet on which you hang your clothes. If the pole was pulled out your clothes would fall into a heap. Your entire system, like the hanging clothes, in certain areas would be completely disrupted.

world seems to be crashing down. Individuals may feel that they no longer have any control over their actions — they become impulsive, haphazard, disconnected from their family and friends. The limbic system seems to run wild and the injured cerebral cortex cannot keep in balance the vast emotions that show (or do not show) themselves. As thinking, feeling, and moving beings if we are not in balance, our actions may bring us only further complications.

Another group of brain structures that works together as a special system is called the basal ganglia. The four nerve cell clusters of the basal ganglia or "nerve knots" help to handle physical movements by relaying information from the cerebral cortex to the brainstem and cerebellum. Most of all, the basal ganglia center serves as a "checking" system that comes to attention when something is not working properly. An injured or diseased (Parkinson's disease) basal ganglia affects voluntary motor nerves, results in slowness and loss of movement (akinesia), muscular rigidity, and tremor, which can be localized or diffuse. When someone loses his/her balance, the neurons in the basal ganglia respond and tell the muscles to restore lost equilibrium.

Most of all, the basal ganglia center serves as a "checking" system that comes to attention when something is not working properly.

The Cerebellum

The interconnectedness of the brain, as we have seen, is difficult to separate as distinct working units since the brain is a complicated organization of multiple systems. Wedged between the brainstem and the cerebral cortex, hitched to the back of the head is the cerebellum. (Our arm-wrist-ball-hand analogy does not represent the cerebellum here unless you want to glue a pingpong ball to the back of your wrist.) It is about 1/8 of the brain's mass and has its own distinctive arrangement of brain cells. Medieval anatomists called the cerebellum "Arbor vitae," the tree of life, because the layers of cells fan out in a striking foliate pattern. The cerebellum governs our every moment and monitors impulses from our motor and steadiness of our movements. It enables us to develop and store the motor skills to play sports, ride a bike, do aerobics exercises, perform martial arts routines, drive a car, and to train our "mind and body" to accomplish amazing athletic feats. Many athletes who train rigorously over months and years coordinate their movements into "automatic" routines, ways to move without even thinking about what they are doing; responding in milliseconds to an opportunity to score the winning point.

Injury or disease to the cerebellum does not produce muscle weakness or changes in our ability to sense things. A person with a damaged cerebellum may look "drunk" when they walk. The person may not even be able to walk a marked straight line or sit without support. The eye and hand coordination so necessary in life may be disabled to the point that the person cannot even reach out and pick up a glass of water. Or the person's movement may become so awkward that trying to brush one's teeth may result in a crushing blow to their own face. Since the cerebellum is responsible for coordinating muscle tone, posture, and eye/hand movements, damage to the cerebellum can seriously inhibit a person's movement within his/her community. Once common routines like getting dressed, writing your name, and getting from class to class in a school become frustrating and impossible to control.

The Cerebral Cortex

By far the most complicated structural component of the brain is the cerebral cortex, which is made up of the right hemisphere and the left hemisphere - each with four lobes bound by three fissures. As you make a fist out of your hand, the cerebral cortex is represented by your hand and fingers. The cortex is full of wrinkles and folds. In fact, if you take cortex and flatten it out it would be the size of a pillowcase. The wrinkling and folding of the cortex helps us pack much more brain mass into our skulls. It is the fact that we have two brains, two hemispheres, that has lead researchers to marvel at the information processing abilities and differences of the cortex. History abounds with references to the "duality of the mind," but it was not until the 1960s that real strides were made, when Dr. Roger Sperry and Dr. Joseph Bogen gave detailed reports of individuals who had undergone surgery to alleviate seizures by cutting the corpus callosum, a complex band of nerve fibers that exchanges information between the two hemispheres. Soon "right brain — left brain" differences became topics for common discussion. The Bogen/Sperry studies showed that the two hemispheres of the brain, while seeming alike, had their own unique ways of processing information. The right hemisphere was more holistic, visual-spatial, and intuitive while the left hemisphere was more linear, verbal-analytic, and logical. From a geographical perspective, comparing the two hemispheres is like comparing the two halves of the United States. They have a major river, the Mississippi, running between them (like the corpus callosum) that serves as a major divider and connector at the same time. While they have similar "rules and regulations," they also have their own distinct styles. The similarities and differences between Californians and New Yorkers exemplifies this. Interestingly, the cerebral hemispheres control opposite sides of the body, thus if a person receives an injury to the right hemisphere he or she will have difficulty controlling their left arm or leg.

According to modern brain scanning, electroencephalograph research, and studies of people who have had their hemispheres separated by surgically sectioning the corpus callosum, the left and right hemispheres demonstrate some processing differences as well as many similarities. The left hemisphere processes information in a logical and linear manner which helps it better understand and use language (speaking, reading, writing, calculations), while the right hemisphere responds to information in a more holistic and spatial sense (shapes, faces, music, art). It is not that the right hemisphere cannot use language. Simple words like book or dog are recognized, but words of higher conceptual demand, like honesty or perseverance, are more difficult. The uniqueness in our cerebral hemispheres is that they do communicate to each other a thousand times per second through the corpus callosum. This four-inch long, pencil thick band of complex nerve fibers allows our two hemispheres to work in tandem. When a student sustains a brain injury the swelling or impact may seriously damage this precious relay system and result in impaired processing of information. Students can have major damage to one hemisphere plus have damage to the corpus callosum pathway. Such injuries create very complex cognitive difficulties for people and many compensatory strategies need to be developed to help rehabilitate people.

In order to more fully understand the impact of an injury to the brain, we need to remember that when one part of the brain is impacted, it reverberates throughout the brain like shock waves through our jello mold. Students with brain injuries will not appear as "one sided" people who have had a stroke in a particular hemisphere. Each brain injury manifests itself differently depending on the type and severity of injury and the age of the student. Children before the age of ten, for example, may sustain an injury which effects their speech center in the left hemisphere, yet these children may be able to develop speech in the opposite area in the right hemisphere. This does not mean that language will progress normally since speech is only one small part of a child's overall language functioning.

We also need to look more closely at the role of the four lobes — frontal, parietal, temporal, and occipital — to better understand the effects of an injury. Because we have two hemispheres our lobes comprise both a left-side and a right-side involvement. Thus, we have a left frontal lobe and right

> When a student sustains a brain injury the swelling or impact may seriously damage this precious relay system and result in impaired processing of information.

frontal lobe, each working together, yet displaying many processing differences just like our hemispheres. These four lobes or areas of brain anatomy are named after the main skull bone that covers it. These landmarks help us to map the surface of the brain, but our lobes do not necessarily match brain areas designated for different tasks. Like the hemispheres with its corpus callosum, our lobes are interconnected by complex neural fibers. The projection fibers fan out from the brainstem and relay impulses and information to and from the cortex. The association fibers loop and link together different sections of the same hemisphere and modulate the cerebral cortex. These two neural fiber systems help the four lobes of our cortex work together and keep it connected intricately with both the limbic system and our brainstem.

The frontal lobe includes everything in front of the central fissure. It is particularly vulnerable to injury since it sits in the front of the skull. The frontal lobe also has extensive connections with the limbic system (emotions) and the other brain lobes. When it is injured or damaged many of a student's abilities are severely compromised, such as the ability to synthesize signals from the environment, assign priorities, make decisions, initiate actions, control emotions, behave and interact socially, make plans, and other executive-like functions. While injury to any designated part of the brain creates problems, injury to the frontal lobe is especially debilitating since the frontal cortex is where ideas are initiated and these ideas have to "go" someplace. It is as if our entire personality changes. A person does not seem to be "like" the person they once were. Our prefrontal cortex in particular is responsible for various emotional responses we have to circumstances. Rather than just responding to situations intellectually, we may respond with delight, anxiety, hope, pessimism, or a range of other higher level emotions.

Frontal lobe injuries in young children often go unnoticed since the children are at an age when caregivers in a sense become their frontal lobes — as teachers and parents we organize, plan, and direct our children's lives. Yet, as the child gets older and enters early adolescence the need for more independent frontal lobe functioning has been diminished by the earlier injury. Students may begin to experience a lack of control over a wide range of behaviors not because they are misbehaving, but because their frontal cortex is not responding normally. Attempts to merely discipline or punish children with frontal lobe injuries does not help them understand or compensate for their loss. Ways to deal with complex behaviors need to be taught to students just like new learning or memory strategies would be introduced.

Spanning our brain like earphones are two adjacent bands of cortex that trigger movement (motor cortex) and register sensations (somatic sensory cortex). This motorsensory strip connecting the frontal and parietal lobes controls every voluntary movement from the simple pointing of a finger to coordinating our lips and tongue to make sounds. The parietal lobe caps the top of the brain behind the central fissure and merges into the occipital lobe. The parietal lobe is the "touchy, feely" part of the brain that responds to touch, heat, cold, pain, and body awareness. Injury to the parietal lobe can cause a loss of these sensing abilities. A student with damage to the right side of the parietal lobe may not even recognize that anything is even wrong with movement of the left side of his/her body, not out of psychological denial but basic neurology. Even more complex functions like attention can be effected by damage to the parietal lobe. The interconnectedness of the brain can impact our motivational states. For example, when we smell food and turn our visual attention (eye movement) towards the source and respond by moving toward the food a complex array of responses are generated through the limbic system, to the frontal lobe, to the parietal lobe, and so on. There are also nerve cells extending as far down as the brain stem to provide the necessary movement and motivational states. Students with injured parietal lobes will experience a host of complex problems in their sensory-motion systems.

The occipital lobe is our primary visual center, yet it is positioned as far away from our eyes as possible in the back of our skull. This explains why when you fall and hit the back of your head, you will oftentimes see "stars" — in effect you have stimulated your occipital lobe. Our visual cortex is connected to our eyes by our optic nerves. No other sense involves so many nerve cells. Vision, neurologically speaking is a complex process. As incoming light rays pass through our eyes and are changed into electrochemical impulses, nerve fibers arrange and code these impulses. Near the back of the eyes, the optic nerves carrying these signals meet at a "crossing" called the optic chiasma. At this cross-point, optic fibers from the inner half of each retina cross to the opposite hemisphere of the brain. Thus, the left optic track carries signals from our right-side field of vision, and the right optic track takes signals from the left so that both sides of our brains in a sense "see" the same thing.

After these signals pass through a relay station in the thalamus and reach the left and right occipital cortex, the whole image is re-assembled and processed by different visual areas for size, shape, position, recognition, color, etc. Most of what we "see" derives its meaning and significance from what it means to us, prior learnings and symbolic representations. And like other areas of the brain, to separate vision from movement, sound, or anything else does not really describe vision in its broadest sense. Unfortunately, injury to the brain often disrupts "what we see" because the complexity of this sense. Visual-perceptual-motoric damage can create many problems for students.

The temporal lobes rest on both sides of the brain and are the centers for language, hearing, and possibly where memories are permanently stored. More than a century ago a French surgeon, Paul Brocca, and a German neurologist, Karl Wernicke, discovered that damage to particular areas of the left temporal and parietal lobes left people unable to speak or unable to understand language. The so-called Brocca's area of the brain is located in the lower portion of the motor cortex in the left frontal-temporal lobe. This area controls muscles of the face and mouth and enables the production of speech. Wernicke's area in the left temporal-parietal lobe governs our understanding of speech and our ability to make sense of our thoughts when we speak. Together these two areas direct the smooth transfer of thought and expression into speech.

The process of hearing, like vision, is very complicated but also different. As sound waves are picked up and passed through our outer and middle ear to our inner ear, a series of events take place. The transmitted sound waves vibrate thousands of tiny sensitive hairs in the organ of Corti. Each hair is connected to thousands of nerve fibers which send signals through the eighth cranial (acoustic) nerve to our brainstem. There, many of the nerve fibers cross over before taking signals up to the tops of our temporal lobes for analysis. A brain injury can produce a breakdown of this process either neurologically or mechanically. While many "mechanical" disruptions to the outer and middle ear can be restructured, damage to the inner ear and temporal lobe can produce more serious consequences.

The memory processing and storage capacities of the temporal lobes are not entirely understood. While the brain can store short-term memories in the hippocampus, long-term memories seem to be holistically stored throughout the brain. The temporal lobes with their connections to the hippocampus may help in this long-term storage of permanent memories in terms of their meaning, retaining concepts and relationships, instead of just words themselves. Students with brain injuries

The temporal lobes rest on both sides of the brain and are the centers for language, hearing, and possibly where memories are permanently stored.

often have difficulty with new learning while exhibiting a good memory for information learned previous to the injury. Their memory system for understanding, storing, and/or retrieving new information has been disrupted by the injury to their brains. When attention, concentration, and memory problems go hand-in-hand, the student will be unable to connect new learnings with prior knowledge and their academic work will seriously suffer.

Recovery and Continued Neurologic Development

The recovery from brain injury is as unique as the injury itself and the child as an individual. Different injuries have different rates and degrees of recovery. A child who experiences a lack of oxygen to his/her brain (i.e., near drowning, strangulation, suffocation, smoke inhalation, cardiac arrest, etc.) tends to have a slow rate of recovery and, depending on the severity of the brain damage, varying prognosis for good recovery. A child who sustains a penetrating head injury (i.e., gunshot wound) may have a more rapid recovery and again, depending on severity, have varying prognosis for recovery.

Professionals commonly use the Rancho Los Amigos Levels Cognitive Functioning (I-VIII) to measure the degree of recovery. The Rancho Levels of Consciousness scales provided below are for infants, 6 month to 2 years; 2-5 year olds; and 5 years and older; and for older adolescents and adults.

Professionals commonly use the Rancho Los Amigos Levels Cognitive Functioning (I-VIII) to measure the degree of recovery.

Rancho Los Amigos Cognitive Scales

Level of Consciousness Records – Head Trauma Patients

Infants, 6 Months to 2 Years

Level I: Interacts with Environment
a) Shows active interest in toys; manipulates or examines before mouthing or discarding.
b) Watches other children at play; may move toward them purposefully.
c) Initiates social contact with adults; enjoys socializing
d) Shows active interest in bottle.
e) Reaches or moves toward person or object.

Level II: Demonstrates Awareness of Environment
a) Responds to name.
b) Recognizes mother or other family members.
c) Enjoys imitative vocal play.
d) Giggles or smiles when talked to or played with.
e) Fussing is quieted by soft voice or touch.

Level III: Gives Localized Response to Sensory Stimuli
a) Blinks when strong light crosses field of vision.
b) Follows moving object passed within visual field.
c) Turns toward or away from loud sound.
d) Gives localized response to painful stimuli.

Level IV: Gives Generalized Response to Sensory Stimuli
a) Gives generalized startle to loud sound.
b) Responds to repeated auditory stimulation with increased or decreased activity.
c) Gives generalized reflex response to painful stimuli.

Level V: No Response to Stimuli
a) Complete absence of observable change in behavior to visual, auditory or painful stimuli.

Preschool – 2 to 5 Years

Level I: Oriented to Self and Surroundings
a) Provides accurate information about self.
b) Knows he is away from home.
c) Knows where toys, clothes, etc., are kept.
d) Actively participates in treatment program.
e) Recognizes own room, knows way to bathroom, nursing station, etc.
f) Is potty trained.
g) Initiates social contact with adult. Enjoys socializing.

Level II: Is Responsive to Environment
a) Follows simple commands.
b) Refuses to follow commands by shaking head or saying "no".
c) Imitates examiner's gestures or facial expressions.
d) Responds to name.
e) Recognizes mother or other family members.
f) Enjoys imitative vocal play.

Level III: Gives Localized Response to Sensory Stimuli
a) Blinks when strong light crosses field of vision.
b) Follows moving object passed within visual field.
c) Turns toward or away from loud sound.
d) Gives localized response to painful stimuli.

Level IV: Gives Generalized Response to Sensory Stimuli
a) Gives generalized startle to loud sound.
b) Responds to repeated auditory stimulation with increased or decreased activity.
c) Gives generalized reflex response to painful stimuli.

Level V: No Response to Stimuli
a) Complete absence of observable change in behavior to visual, auditory or painful stimuli.

While we have certainly begun to discover how our brains work, we have only scratched the surface of our neurological wonders. The brain is certainly the most precious and complicated organ in our body.

School Age – 5 Years & Older

**Level I: Oriented to Time & Place:
Is Recording Ongoing Events**
a) Can provide accurate, detailed information about self and present situation.
b) Knows way to and from daily activities.
c) Knows sequence of daily routine.
d) Knows way around unit; recognizes own room.
e) Can find own bed; knows where personal belongings are kept.
f) Is bowel and bladder trained.

Level II: Is Responsive to Environment
a) Follows simple verbal or gestured requests.
b) Initiates purposeful activity.
c) Actively participates in therapy program.
d) Refuses to follow request by shaking head or saying "no".
e) Imitates examiner's gestures or facial expressions.

Level III: Gives Localized Response to Sensory Stimuli
a) Blinks when strong light crosses field of vision.
b) Follows moving object passed within visual field.
c) Turns toward or away from loud sound.
d) Gives localized response to painful stimuli.

Level IV: Gives Generalized Response to Sensory Stimuli
a) Gives generalized startle to loud sound.
b) Responds to repeated auditory stimulation with increased or decreased activity.
c) Gives generalized reflex response to painful stimuli.

Level V: No Response to Stimuli
a) Complete absence of observable change in behavior to visual, auditory or painful stimuli.

Adult Rancho Los Amigos Cognitive Scale

Level I
No response to pain, touch, sound, or sight.

Level II
Generalized reflex response to pain.

Level III
Localized response. Blinks to strong light, turns toward/away from sound, responds to physical discomfort, inconsistent response to commands.

Level IV
Confused–Agitated. Alert, very active, aggressive or bizarre behaviors, performs motor activities but behavior is non-purposeful, extremely short attention span.

Level V
Confused–Non-agitated. Gross attention to environment, highly distractible, requires continual redirection, difficulty learning new tasks, agitated by too much stimulation. May engage in social conversation but with inappropriate verbalizations.

Level VI
Confused–Appropriate. Inconsistent orientation to time and place, retention span/recent memory impaired, begins to recall past, consistently follows simple directions, goal-directed behavior with assistance.

Level VII
Automatic–Appropriate. Performs daily routines in highly familiar environment in a non-confused but automatic robot-like manner. Skills noticeably deteriorate in unfamiliar environment. Lacks realistic planning for own future.

Level VIII
Purposeful–Appropriate.

Many educators will see that the Rancho Levels of Consciousness scales for children are assessing the child's awareness of and interaction with the environment, the child's orientation to self, other people and surroundings, and responses to sensory stimuli. Such assessments are not unlike many of the developmental inventories that educators use to evaluate children. The difference is that a child with a brain injury is "recovering" from a specific event in time and their injury has implications for the child's immediate needs as well as his/her continued development over time.

Thus, a brain injury to a child may be very different when compared with a brain injury to an adult, even when the exact same areas/systems of the brain have been damaged. A child's brain is still growing and developing, thus, an injury to a child's brain in the early years may not exhibit the same or as serious an array of problems as a similar injury might with an adult. Unfortunately, as the child develops and matures, earlier brain injuries can create later problems. A baby who falls and injures the frontal lobes of his/her brain may appear very normal in the ensuing years. However, as the child approaches puberty and the frontal lobes are being called on more and more to handle the complexities of life, the child's previously injured brain may not respond as it normally should. When we look at brain injury in children we need to look at it from a developmental perspective.

Brain growth during development inside the womb and in the five years after birth is extremely accelerated when compared to other parts of the body. A newborn baby's brain has reached one quarter of its adult weight although the baby is only one twentieth as heavy as the adult he/she will become. Prebirth growth of the brain results from cells multiplying in the brain in a series of "supports." After birth the baby's brain grows not only in weight, but in complexity. Yet, even though the newborn baby's brain has almost all the neurons his/her brain will ever hold, the newborn baby has yet to form the connections and systems that develop the brain into an organized and integrated organ. This is an especially important point to note when discussing injury to infants and toddlers. It is difficult to assess the extent of damage to children who have been abused, fallen, or have been injured in motor vehicle crashes since their brain is still so immature. However, early damage to an already underdeveloped and immature brain does not mean that the child will just "grow out of it". The often held notion of brain plasticity and ability to rebound from serious injury does no necessarily hold true when it comes to the brain. Consequently, children who have been badly shaken and/or struck by a parent, or have sustained a blow to the head in a car crash or a fall may end up with long term neurologic problems that may become more complicated over time.

Developmentally parallel to this is the concern about children who sustain brain injuries at other ages and what happens to those children over time. Many educators, pediatricians, psychologists and child life specialists have presented the concept that children and youth are "developing" over time. Children are not merely miniature adults, but are beings in their own right with their own wants and needs. Unfortunately, many of the measurement instruments we use to assess brain injury, while developed for adults, are commonly used with children. Many of these measurement tools give us a false impression of the child's injury and needs.

The critical issues of brain growth and development and subsequent injury to a child's brain are areas in need of in-depth and long-term study. While we have certainly begun to discover how our brains work, we have only scratched the surface of our neurological wonders. The brain is certainly the most precious and complicated organ in the body. Quite simply our brain is who we are and who we will become. When the brain of a child is injured it can become a life-time experience which deeply effects the child and the family.

An understanding of the brain and what happens when it is injured will help educators better plan their teaching strategies and materials. Knowing how the brain develops, grows, and works will enable us to develop educational plans that can focus on the strengths and needs of children as they continue their lives.

References

Brown, C. (1977). *Mechanics of the mind.* New York: Cambridge University Press.

Epstein, H. (1979). Growth spurts during brain development: Implications for educational policy. In J. Chall (Ed.), *Education and the brain: National Society for the Study of Education Yearbook.* Chicago: University of Chicago Press.

Hart, L.A. (1975). *How the brain works.* New York: Basic Books.

Hart, L.A. (1983). *Human brain and human learning.* New York: Longman.

Harth, E. (1982). *Windows on the mind: Reflections on the physical basis of consciousness.* New York: Morrow.

Lambert, D., Bramwell, M., & Lawther, G. (Eds.). (1987). *The brain: A user's manual* (2nd ed.). New York: G.P. Putnam's Sons.

Luria, A.R. (1973). *The working brain: An introduction to neuropsychology.* New York Penguin Press.

Restak, R.M. (1979). *The brain: The last frontier.* New York: Doubleday.

Restak, R. (1984). *The brain.* New York: Bantam.

Restak, R. (1986). *The infant mind.* New York: Doubleday.

Restak, R. (1988). *The mind.* New York: Bantam.

Restak, R. (1991) *The brain has a mind of its own.* New York: Harmony Books.

Taylor, G.R. (1979). *The natural history of the mind.* New York: Dutton.

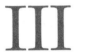

Creating a Workable Education Program

BETH URBANCZYK, M.S.CCC-SLP
RONALD C. SAVAGE, ED.D.
ROBERTA DEPOMPEI, PH.D., CCC-SLP/A
JEAN L. BLOSSER, ED.D., CCC-SLP

Focus:
Planning for School Entry and Reintegration
Transition Planning
Designing the IEP and Transition Plan
Creating an Effective Classroom Environment

Despite the many brain injury rehabilitation programs in this country, our public schools are still the largest provider of services for individuals with brain injury (Ylvisaker, Hartwick, & Stevens, 1991; Savage, 1991). In fact, returning to school is one of the primary goals for children and adolescents following brain injury. Presently, in our school systems there are three major issues facing students and their families following brain injury: how to best identify and classify such individuals under federal and state special education laws; how best to transition these students back into their school systems; and how to best monitor and plan their academic programs. These educational issues are critical to the long-term success of students with brain injuries and their eventual transition into the adult world of work and community living. Students with brain injuries returning to their schools may come from an acute care hospital, a short-term rehabilitation program, a long-term rehabilitation facility, or home. Unfortunately, the majority of students with brain injuries will be discharged directly home from the acute care hospital. According to the National Pediatric Trauma Registry (DiScala 1993), brain injury was the most frequent diagnosis among children recorded in the registry. According to the registry, 93% of the children admitted to trauma centers are discharged home. Referrals for outpatient services, such as, physical and occupational therapy and speech/language therapy were limited for children that demonstrated at least one functional limitation at the time of discharge. Recommendations for special education services were made for less than 2% of these children. This places a great burden on the educational system to not only accurately identify these students, but to plan an appropriate educational program to meet the many needs of a student with a brain injury. For those students returning from acute care hospitals, their time away from school will probably number only a few days or weeks and they will have available a restricted range of professional reports (neurology/neurosurgery, physical/occupational therapy, speech/language therapy) that may be utilized to update school staff. Students who are discharged from short-term rehabilitation facilities generally have experienced a more substantial disruption of their academic and social lives. They may also demonstrate more severe impairments of learning and communication skills. School personnel should expect more complete information regarding the child's ability to function within a school setting from a short-term rehabilitation program. A comprehensive neuropsychological evaluation should be made available to school personnel from the majority of short-term rehabilitation programs. Students returning from long-term rehabilitation facilities, such as residential or day treatment programs, may have ongoing needs for intensive rehabilitation interventions and may have been separated from their friends and home school for months or years. Long-term facilities should provide school personnel with thorough and accurate descriptions of the child's abilities and areas of need, as well as a copy of the educational plan implemented at that facility.

Lastly, for those students who return to school from home, there is often little information available about the severity of their injury and the educational interventions and environmental modifications they may need. Students with brain injuries may return to school from a variety of circumstances and with a multitude of needs. The transition from a hospital, rehabilitation center, or home to school is a key factor in the long-term success of a child with a brain injury.

Planning for School Re-Integration

Public Law 101-476 now enables school systems to better identify the needs of students with brain injury. Schools and teachers across the country have been and are still receiving training about brain injury and the needs of these students in order to better provide regular and special education services. Many states have set up interdisciplinary teams to develop programs to help students with

(sidebar) **Students who are discharged from short-term rehabilitation facilities generally have experienced a more substantial disruption of their academic and social lives. They may also demonstrate more severe impairments of learning and communication skills.**

brain injuries in their ongoing recovery. Essential to this process is the ability of the initial health care provider and the school system to collaborate when the child or adolescent is still in the early stages of recovery.

The return to school can be devastating if the health care facility (hospital or rehabilitation center) and the student's home school do not interact as soon as possible and as frequently as possible (Savage, 1984, Carter & Savage, 1988; DePompei & Blosser, 1987; Blosser & DePompei, 1989; Blosser & DePompei, 1994; Ylvisaker, Hartwick, & Stevens, 1991, Begali, 1992; Mira et al., 1992; Lash, 1992). The inclusion of brain injury in our special education laws has helped to improve our understanding of the medical and educational needs of children and adolescents. Hence, as soon as a student is admitted to a health care facility (hospital and/or rehabilitation center), the school reintegration and transition process needs to start. Transition of the student with brain injury into the educational system is not a one-time process. It is a process that will continue throughout the child's academic career.

> The inclusion of brain injury in our special education laws has helped to improve our understanding of the medical and educational needs of children and adolescents.

Experience has demonstrated that successful school reintegration and transition needs to involve six basic steps:

1. involvement of the school-based special and regular education team in the hospital or rehabilitation facility;
2. involvement of the child's long term medical team (pediatrician, neurologist, etc) in the hospital, rehabilitation facility and with the school-based education team;
3. inservice training for all school-based staff who will have contact with the child;
4. information sharing with friends and peers of the student with brain injury;
5. short and long term program planning for the student's IEP.;
6. continued follow-up by the rehabilitation professionals.

(Savage & Carter, 1988)

Blosser & DePompei (1994) developed a checklist that can be used by educators, rehabilitation specialists, and families to effectively plan for school reentry (Table 6-1). This checklist can be employed during initial planning meetings and during transitions.

Action to be Taken Person/s Responsible Date

I. Prior to Returning to School

A. Identify one individual at each facility who will serve as liaison and coordinator of networking. (Make the decision jointly with family.)

B. Follow all established school policies and procedures for exchanging information and communicating with other agencies.

C. Schedule a meeting to discuss plans for the student. Invite family members and people who have been involved with the student's rehabilitation as well as former and new educators.

D. Compile as much information about the student as possible based on comments from family and friends, test data, and observations.

E. Establish a plan for exchanging information, educating one another, and developing an effective reintegration plan.

F. Learn about the student's present status (including impairments, strengths, needs, interests).

1. Obtain medical/rehabilitation records.

2. Find out about the medical aspects of the injury (nature and extent of damage).

3. Construct a record treatment history and progress.

4. Generate a profile characterizing the student's skills and capabilities as well as needs at the time of reintegration. Be prepared to update frequently as changes occur.

5. Identify the physical, cognitive-communicative, and social behaviors that are likely to interfere with learning and social activities at school.

6. Obtain samples of the student's work that are representative of current capabilities and levels of performance.

G. Relate information gained to the general requisite needs for educational success.

1. Discuss characteristics of the school and various class settings, expectations for performance, routines, learning materials, classmates, and so on.

2. Determine the student's readiness to participate in school activities based on the recognized demands of the educational setting.

3. Discuss options and educational choices available to the student. Strive for a high level of inclusion.

H. Evaluate the school's readiness and capabilities for meeting the student's needs at the time.1. Discuss applicable school policies and procedures regarding meeting a student's special needs (including special education and related service options, eligibility criteria, staff capabilities, and so on.)

2. Make arrangements for pertinent assessments to obtain information for educational planning.

3. Determine obstacles that may interfere with successful reintegration. Look at the student critically from the perspective of program offerings, personnel, and so on.

4. Search for the most appropriate class selection and personnel.

5. Determine how to modify, eliminate, or reduce the obstacles. Establish objectives (for the environment, the educators, the student).

I. Search for the most appropriate class and personnel to meet the student's needs. Consider several critical elements:

1. Review the instructional objectives associated with the selected class.

2. Determine if the objectives are compatible with the student's capabilities and long-term needs.

3. Analyze the socialization characteristics, demands, and needs.

4. Observe the classroom climate and environment.

5. Evaluate the teacher's willingness to learn and/or level of understanding of youngster's with TBI.

6. Determine if key educator characteristics are present including: flexibility, acceptance, patience, positive, supportive attitude, competence, and repertoire of teaching techniques.

J. Prepare an Individualized Education Plan (IEP) addressing the student's needs and confirming specific recommendations for modification of the environment and techniques educators and others can use to help the student.

II. After the Reintegration

A. Maintain ongoing communication about the student's performance through an organized flow of information.

B. Look ahead to the next stages in the student's educational experience. Determine other educators who will be involved. Formulate a plan for preparing them to meet the student's needs.

C. Develop peer support systems by: educating peers, alerting them to the student's problems and ways for helping, and providing opportunities for involvement in extracurricular activities.

D. Gather family and personnel who have been involved with the student. Summarize the student's performance and the overall success of the reintegration. Discuss satisfaction with learner outcomes.

E. Decide what program aspects can be changed, eliminated, or increased to raise future potential.

F. Prepare a transition plan to enable proactive response to situations to be encountered.

G. Additional Items of Importance

Source: Blosser, J. & DePompei, R. (1994). Pediatric traumatic brain injury: Proactive intervention. San Diego, CA: Singular Publishing Group, Inc.

Referral for Special Education

A designated representative from the hospital and/or rehabilitation facility needs to immediately inform the school that they are presently caring for one of the school's students. The family and/or the attending physician must formally request that the school come in and evaluate the child. The referral is typically made to the Director of Special Education and should include the following information: child's name, date of birth, date of injury, date of admission to hospital and/or rehabilitation facility, mechanism of injury (i.e., motor vehicle collision, fall, bicycle crash, etc), name(s) of family member and/or physician making the referral, the federal and state regulations for brain injury, as well as a stated commitment by the hospital and/or rehabilitation facility to be an active partner in the school reintegration process for the student. This letter should be copied to the principal of the child's home school to ensure that all the key players are included in planning for the child's return to school. Blosser and DePompei provide a worksheet format for team review and analysis of pertinent information (Figure 3-2, following).

Initial Contact:

The initial contact between the school-based team and the hospital and/or rehabilitation team is important as it can set the tone for the entire transition process. It is a time for both systems to begin to understand each other and how to blend their areas of expertise into a plan that will give the child the best chance to succeed in school and at home.

The hospital-based team typically includes: a physician (neurologist, physiatrist, pediatrician, etc), a primary care nurse, a service coordinator, a speech/language pathologist, a physical therapist and a physical therapy assistant, an occupational therapist and a certified occupational therapy assistant, a social worker/rehabilitation counselor, a neuropsychologist, and a therapeutic recreation specialist. Few short-term rehabilitation facilities employ educators. The school-based team typically includes: the director of special education, the principal, regular and special education teachers and aides, a speech/language pathologist, physical and occupational therapists, a school nurse, a school psychologist and a social worker. These two teams of professionals need to identify ways to share information, ways to speak the same "language," and ways to recreate environmental factors that help the child to succeed in both settings. DePompei & Blosser (1993) have suggested a number of methods for developing communication between service providers at rehabilitation and education settings.

At some point during this or another visit, the school-based team should be provided specific information regarding the brain and brain injury, the child's injury and what they can expect now and in the future.

Figure 3-2

Planning Worksheet for Team Review and Analysis

General Status

Each team member should make a statement of his or her observations and impressions of the student's general behavior and status.

Medical Status

Area of brain involved: _____

Severity of injury: _____

Extent of motoric involvement: _____

Glasgow Coma Scale: _____

Ranchos Los Amigos Level:

_____ At Discharge

_____ At School Reentry

_____ 3 Months Post Injury

_____ 6 Months Post Injury

_____ 9 Months Post Injury

Seizure Activity: _____

Medication: _____

Type: _____ Dosage: _____

Health status at time of reintegration: _____

Potential impact of medical status on intervention:

_____

_____

_____

_____

_____

_____

_____

_____

Cognitive-Communication Status

(Based on test results and observations)

Expressive Language	Receptive Language
Phonology	Orientation
Syntax	Attention
Semantics	Memory
Pragmatics	Association
	Executive Functioning

Psychosocial Status

Interpersonal behaviors with family, friends:

_____

Mood most days

_____

Potential impact of psychosocial behavior on intervention:

_____

_____

_____

Academic Information

Grade level in specific curricular areas *(math, reading, language arts, writing)*

_____

Strengths and needs in classroom related behaviors *(attending, self control, awareness, independence, persistence, organization, problem solving, information processing)*

_____

_____

_____

Source: From "A Proactive Model for Treating Communication Disorders in Children and Adolescents with Traumatic Brain Injury" by J. Blosser and R. DePompei, 1992, Clinics in Communication Disorders, 2, p. 56. Copyright 1992 by Elsevier Science, Inc. Reprinted by permission.

Visits to the Hospital and School:

At least once during the child's inpatient hospitalization, select members of the child's school-based team should observe the child during his/her interactions with his/her rehabilitation team. If only one or two members of the school-based team are available to visit, it is best to have one member that will work with the child on a daily basis and one member from "administration" that will be available to follow the child as he/she transitions from grade to grade. This visit, along with the requested evaluation are the important first steps in initiating the special education process for identification and classification purposes (i.e., does this student need special education services and how should he/she best be classified). During the visit to the rehabilitation facility, the school-based team should have an opportunity to meet the child and family, observe the student in therapy, have an opportunity to discuss the sequelae of brain injury as it relates to this child specifically and in general, and have an opportunity to meet with the rehabilitation team. This allows members of the rehabilitation team to share the various rehabilitation techniques, materials, and assessment instruments being utilized. It also allows the two teams time to clarify terminology utilized by their respective systems that may be confusing. The designated representative from the hospital and/or rehabilitation facility should gather and provide the school with information in a written and/or visual format in regards to recovery prognosis, school reintegration, possible sequelae as a result of brain injury, cognitive/communicative issues following brain injury and challenging behaviors following brain injury, etc.

It is equally as important for members of the hospital-based team to visit the school as it is for the school-based team to visit the rehabilitation center. During this visit, the member(s) of the hospital-based team should have ample opportunity to sit down with all members of the child's school-based team in order to discuss specific concerns regarding the child's health, behavior, means of communication and learning issues. It is also a time to discuss a potential schedule: what lunch period would be best; how is the child going to get from point A to point B; what height should the desk be; and what time of day is best for math, etc. At some point during this or another visit, the school-based team should be provided specific information regarding the brain and brain injury, the child's injury and what they can expect now and in the future. It is also crucial that information is shared with the child's peers. This can be presented in several different ways. The child and a member of the rehabilitation team can do a co-presentation; a member of the rehabilitation team can bring a videotape of the child, provide information to the peers and then show the videotape, or a designated member of the school-based team can be the designated person for the other students to contact to discuss the child's current status, to discuss their feelings regarding the child's injury or to just ask questions. Regardless of the method of presentation, peers must be included in the student's return to school.

Developing the IEP:

Once the school has determined that the student is in need of special education services and has appropriately identified the child as a student with brain injury, then the school can begin to develop the Individual Education Plan (IEP). For those students 16 years and older, individual transition plans also need to be developed, as well as for those students under age 16 years if deemed appropriate and necessary.

The IEP is essentially the "negotiated contract" between the child's family and the school system regarding the kinds and extent of services the student needs (Carter & Savage, 1988; Ylvisaker et al., 1991). DePompei and Blosser (1991) and Blosser DePompei (1994) suggest methods for directly involving the family in the IEP process. They describe the family's roles and responsibilities as well as guidance service providers can give.

In the case of the student whose brain injury is mild, full-fledged special education programming may not be immediately necessary. Those students may only need to be monitored or have their schedules modified for a period of time to insure that any neurologic sequela has resolved. If not, the school nurse, classroom teachers, and family can then alert the child's physician and/or neuropsychologist to any persistent problems the student may be experiencing.

In the case of students with more severe injuries, both medical and educational professionals need to recognize that school reintegration is best facilitated by coordinated systems of care, rather than merely passing the child from one institution to another. Developing communication protocols between health care facilities, school systems and families will help eliminate the "cracks" between systems to which all too many children and their families fall victim.

Thus, the initial IEP should be a "joint venture" among the health care facility, the school, and the family. This initial IEP can reflect the cognitive, psychosocial, and neuromotor needs of the student from a functionally-based and process-centered approach that will enable the student to become increasingly more involved in his/her school, family, and community as he/she continues to recover.

For example, consider a student with a brain injury who is back in school but is experiencing difficulty remembering historical dates and facts in his/her social studies class. This student may need his/her work area in the classroom restructured to enhance concentration and attention and use specific memory strategies to help store and retrieve information. Such therapeutic interventions that worked well in the rehabilitation setting can be carried over into the school setting and these strategies need to be shared with the family so they can be continued at home. Collaborative planning that starts early in the rehabilitation setting and can be extended into school helps merge the health care and school systems with the family into a unified, ongoing program. Again, the IEP is driven by federal mandate and is the best vehicle we have to negotiate and agree to service delivery models which are in the best interests of the student.

Another important component in the IEP process is the duration of the educational plan. Many IEPs are written to serve other children with special needs through an entire school year. For many children with brain injuries, needs change dramatically as they recover or experience emotional/behavioral changes. Therefore, it is wise to create IEPs that are not bound by artificial time-barriers. Writing an IEP for a child with a brain injury and not re-evaluating the student or the IEP for the entire academic year can have grave consequences. Students and their individual education plans need to be reviewed frequently to coincide with changes in recovery. Students with brain injuries, unlike other students with diagnosed developmental or learning disabilities, often continue to make remarkable changes in the first year following the injury. Thus, the IEP needs to incorporate frequent review times to monitor progress or potential problems.

First IEP: Student Still in a Hospital

After the child's eligibility for special education services has been determined, the first IEP can be developed prior to the child's return to school. The initial IEP can specify:

1. Goals/objectives to be pursued in the medical facility by the hospital-based team;
2. Responsibility for assessment in relation to school re-entry (e.g., who should do the mandatory

testing?) How can functional academically-oriented assessments be conducted in the medical facility so that school staff have educationally relevant information prior to the return of the student?

3. The school's responsibilities prior to the return of the student;

a. Monitoring the student's progress and communicating with the medical facility;

b. Preparing relevant staff once a placement decision has been made; (e.g. visit to the hospital; inservice training; identification of useful readings for teacher preparation; team formation.)

First School IEP:

1. Duration: With many children with brain injuries, needs change dramatically as they recover or experience emotional/behavioral changes. Therefore, it is wise to create IEPs that are not bound by artificial time-barriers. Students with brain injuries, unlike other students with diagnosed developmental or learning disabilities, often continue to make remarkable changes in the first year following the injury. Thus, the IEP needs to incorporate frequent review times to monitor progress or potential problems.

2. Team Formation: The initial IEP should specify team process issues. There should be regular team meetings led by a designated Team Leader/Service Coordinator. These team meetings are particularly important in the early weeks and months after return to school — and again at transitional times. During these team meetings, progress and problems will be identified and solutions proposed.

3. Contingencies for Program Changes: Students and their individual education plans need to be reviewed frequently to coincide with changes in recovery. It is not easy to know what program will be best when a student returns from a hospital. Therefore, it is important to specify criteria for changing the student's program. For example, what criteria must be met for a student to add additional components of an academic program? What criteria must be met to add more regular education components?

4. Time Frames: It is well to specify anticipated time frames for program changes, so that staff are alert to the need to raise these issues in a timely manner.

5. Identify Program Goals/Activities that are Relevant to Same Age/Same Grade Peers: It is essential to work within the student's ability level, but also within the general context of age-appropriate material and activities.

6. Capacity (versus Deficit) Focus: This is connected with the necessity of identifying a student's remaining capacities, even in cases in which deficits abound. As much as possible, programming should be conceived as building on capacities, versus simply attempting to remediate deficits.

7. Psychosocial Goals: Anticipating the very common evolution of isolation and depression over the months after return to school, staff should address these issues proactively by:

a. Ensuring that there are some activities in school at which the student can succeed/excel;

b. Trying to identify a circle of friends for emotional support.

8. Long-Term Focus: It is important to consider long-term issues that are common for this group of students (i.e., continued recovery and neurologic development, vocational planning, home/community transitions, etc.). This is especially important in light of the growing body of literature that is focusing on the long-term developmental issues associated with brain injury in childhood.

9. Family Involvement: Families tend to be the only ones who have seen and followed this child from the day of the injury to the day the child returns to school. The family is the expert on that

The creation of an effective classroom environment for a student with a brain injury necessarily involves all the individuals that will spend time with the child at any point during his/her day, family members, and a representative from the hospital/rehabilitation center.

child and as such, they should be actively involved in the development of the IEP. Siblings' needs should be considered and possible supports or services provided. And their needs as a family should be considered and possible supports or services provided.

10. Inclusion in General Education Classroom: There is currently an effort to increase inclusion for students with varying educational disabilities. Inclusion is a particularly important theme for students returning to school after a brain injury for several reasons:

a. A student is accustomed to this setting and therefore special education settings may be both disorienting and emotionally challenging.

b. A student often improves neurologically after returning to school. Therefore placement that is somewhat beyond his/her current level of performance (with needed supports) may be appropriate.

As in other cases, inclusionary education requires appropriate levels of support and training for the general education teachers.

Summer Transitions:

A student returning home from a hospital/rehabilitation facility over the summer that may require an educational program presents a significant challenge to the educational system. Many school districts are under budget restrictions, provide only summer programming for children with "severe and profound" disabilities, have staffing that is significantly less than during the academic year, and the special education committee is oftentimes a mixture of people that are covering the summer months. These factors, along with the relative newness of the TBI classification, serve to make a summer transition into an educational program challenging for all involved.

During the child's inpatient hospitalization, his/her day is typically highly structured and provides ample opportunity for learning, communicating and improving overall physical abilities. Paired with the reality of decreasing lengths of stay (sometimes as short as 2 - 4 weeks), many children are being discharged home during a period of time in which they are demonstrating rapid improvements in their cognitive abilities, communication abilities and physical abilities. This is a prime time to work with the child in terms of developing compensatory strategies to assist in learning and communicating and how to negotiate this "new world" the child may find himself/herself living in after the injury. The educational programming provided over the summer is essential for the child's successful transition into the academic year. If the child's structured day, and opportunities for learning new information and possibly relearning old information are limited during the summer months the child will more than likely demonstrate regression in terms of learning ability. If the educational program that is developed over the summer is not thoughtfully planned out, the child's first experiences with the school after the injury may be negative and begin a downward spiral that leads to failure and frustration for the child, his/her family, and the school. With open and ongoing communication between the school, the family and the rehabilitation facility, this downward spiral of failure and frustration can be avoided. The authors have had many positive opportunities to develop creative IEPs for summer programs for students with brain injury.

Mild Brain Injury:

Many children return to school after very mild injuries (and sometimes after more severe injuries) with no apparent effects of the injury. If there are to be educational consequences of the injury, they are generally revealed in changed classroom performance as opposed to weakness on formal testing. Therefore, classroom behavior and academic performance should be used as the basic assessment for these students.

If the following behaviors are observed within the first three to four weeks following return to school after mild brain injury, they should be considered "red flags" signalling that possible consequences and accommodations should be put in place to prevent academic and social failure. However, if symptoms of altered ability or performance persist beyond four weeks, referral should be made to the school psychologist for assessment. Red flags include (All of these behaviors must be judged relative to the student's performance before the injury):

1. Attendance: Unexpected absences from school or from specific classes.

2. Academic Performance:
a. Inattentiveness beyond what is normally expected of the student.
b. Academic performance lower than before the injury.
c. Relatively slow performance; delayed responses.
d. Difficulty remembering new information or assignments.

3. Social/Behavioral Performance:
a. Unexpected conflict with peers.
b. Excessive tiredness.
c. Excessive moodiness; unexpected mood swings.

Creating An Effective Classroom Environment

A very wise Committee on Special Education chairperson from upstate New York made the statement, "We need to look at what the student's day needs to look like and from there we will develop his/her IEP." Taking this type of viewpoint enabled the creation of an outstanding educational program that equally valued the classroom environment, and the people that were needed in that environment to help this child succeed. The creation of an effective classroom environment for a student with a brain injury necessarily involves all the individuals that will spend time with the child at any point during his/her day, family members, and a representative from the hospital/rehabilitation center. Although this may initially be cumbersome and time consuming, it is well worth the time and effort required. It is better to pay now, than pay later.

The School Function Assessment developed by Coster, Deeney, Haltiwanger and Haley (Coster et al., 1994) provides an excellent means to look at the child's ability to function within the school. Issues such as: transportation to and from school and within the school building itself; transitions within a class; transitions from class to class; participation in the classroom setting (regular classroom, special education classroom); cafeteria; bathroom; playground; and physical education issues all need to be addressed when developing the classroom/school environment. The education of school staff, students, and other support personnel within the school in regard to brain injury and its consequences is equally important in developing a culture within the school that supports the child's new abilities and challenges following the injury.

Physical modifications to the classroom can be decided upon prior to the child's discharge home. Typical modifications may include: creating aisles that are wheelchair accessible; finding a desk that is the right height and provides proper support; placement of the desk near the teacher or the front of the room, etc. This is an excellent opportunity for collaboration between the teacher and physical and/or occupational therapist.

The most important environmental modifications that occur when creating an effective classroom environment for a child with a brain injury are the modifications of other people's means of interacting with and teaching the child. The people involved with the child may include any or all of the following: the regular education teacher; the special education teacher; a classroom aide; the building principal; the guidance counselor; the school psychologist; the school nurse; the speech/language pathologist; the physical therapist; the occupational therapist; the director of special education; the physical educator/coach; the social worker; the janitor; the lunchroom staff ; and secretarial staff. Specific learning strategies and means of presenting information to the child as well as ways to structure the educational program should be provided to and by the educators (regular and special education) prior to the child's return to school or transition from one grade or school to the next. Modifications may include: having the teacher provide his/her notes to the child from a classroom lecture; audiotaping classroom lectures; repetition and/or restatement of information; providing information in simple, concrete terms that are respectful of the child's age; shortening assignments to the critical pieces of information that must be learned; providing the child with multiple opportunities to learn new information; providing the special education teacher with lesson plans from each class in order to help the child develop/refine strategies to learn; and have a focus on working with the child on learning how to learn versus a focus on mastery of academic content.

As stated earlier, it is important to include the child's friends and peers as part of the environmental modifications. Inclusion of the child's friends and peers in this support system must be evaluated in terms of its helpfulness to the child with a brain injury and the benefit to the peer. Oftentimes, a friend may have been involved in the crash and come away uninjured, which may lead to intense feelings of guilt. He/she may want to become overinvolved in the child's return to school. If a friend wants to volunteer as a peer tutor or to be a part of a circle of friends, it is important to let the child know it is okay if he/she cannot fulfill those obligations. A Student Council organization within the school tends to be an organization that can provide additional support to the child not only academically, but socially as well. The child needs to be involved in extracurricular activities as well to assist with social reintegration. There are many different opportunities within schools for assisting the child with developing and maintaining friendships. The child and his family must have an active role in deciding upon these opportunities. The development and maintenance of friendships is just as much a part of the child's education as is learning multiplication tables. The bottomline when looking at and creating a classroom environment is to create externally what may have been injured internally. This environment may need frequent revisions to keep pace with the child's rate of recovery. It is important to recognize the fact that the program developed initially will change many times throughout the child's academic career.

A final piece to consider when creating an effective classroom environment is readjusting peoples' misconceptions of a child with a brain injury. School staff and other personnel need to understand the child's new abilities and challenges, not provide excuses for the difficulty that may be encountered in educating this child. The staff involved in this child's education will benefit from supporting the concept that the issue of "getting along" socially is just as important as learning facts and figures. Developing an effective classroom environment can be challenging, yet it is only limited by the creativity of those now involved in this child's life.

Bibliography

Blosser, J.L., & DePompei, R. (1994). Creating an effective classroom environment. In R. Savage & G. Wolcott (Eds.) Educational dimensions of acquired brain injury. Austin: Pro-Ed.

Blosser, J.L. & DePompei, R. (1994). Pediatric traumatic brain injury: Proactive Intervention. San Diego, CA: Singular Publishing Group.

Blosser, J. & DePompei, R. (1992). A proactive model for treating communication disorders in children and adolescents with traumatic brain injury. Clinics in Communication Disorders, 2(2), 52-65.

Blosser, J.L., & DePompei, R. (1989). The head injured student returns to school: Recognizing and treating deficits. Topics in Language Disorders, 9, 67-77.

DePompei, R. & Blosser, J.L. (1993). Professional training and development for pediatric rehabilitation. In C. Durgin, N. Schmidt, & J. Freyer (Eds.), Staff development and clinical intervention in brain injury rehabilitation, (pp. 229-253). Gaithersburg, MD: Aspen.

DePompei, R. & Blosser, J. (1991). Families of children with traumatic brain injury as advocates in school reentry. Neurorehabilitation, 1(2), 29-37.

DePompei, R., & Blosser, J.L. (1987). Strategies for helping head-injured children successsfully return to school. Language, Speech, and Hearing Services in Schools, 18, 292- 300.

DiScala, C. (1993). Pediatric Trauma Registry biannual report.Boston: Tufts University, Research and Training Center, National Pediatric Trauma Registry.

Lehr, E., & Savage, R.C. (1990). Community and school integration from a developmental perspective. In Community integration following traumatic brain injury. Baltimore: Brookes.

Mira, M., Tyler, J., & Tucker, B. (1988). Traumatic head injury in children: A guide for schools. Kansas City, KA: University of Kansas Medical Center.

Rosen, C.D., & Gerring, J.P. (1992). Head trauma: Educational reintegration (second edition). San Diego: Singular Press.

Savage, R.C. (1991). Identification, classification, and placement issues for students with traumatic brain injuries.Journal of Head Trauma Rehabilitation, 6, 1-9.

Savage, R.C., & Carter, R.R. (1984). Re-entry: the head injured student returns to school. Cognitive Rehabilitation, 2, 28-33.

Savage, R.C., & Carter, R.R. (1988). Transitioning pediatric patients into educational systems: guideline for rehabilitation professionals. Cognitive Rehabilitation, 6(4).

Savage, R.C., & Mishkin, L. (1994). A neuroeducational model for teaching students with acquired brain injuries. In Educational dimensions of acquired brain injury. Austin: Pro*Ed.

Contributed by Susan Pearson

Allison

In December 1989, when Allison was 14 years old, she experienced a brain injury in a motor vehicle accident. She was in a coma for 18 days and remained in the hospital for approximately two months. A CAT scan at the time of Allison's injury was consistent with diffuse bilateral hemispheric swelling with possible small subarachnoid hemorrhage in the frontal region. At the time of her discharge, she began receiving outpatient therapy services through a local hospital. She did not return to school for the spring semester, but was re-evaluated in June in order to determine what her needs would be for the following school year.

Prior to her head injury, Allison had significant family and behavior/social problems. She had run away from home four times and by age eleven had experimented with both alcohol and drugs. She attended four different elementary schools, missing an average of about ten days each year. In sixth-grade, her attendance was especially poor and she failed all major classes in seventh-grade. She was given the opportunity to go to summer school, but chose to repeat seventh-grade instead. Prior to October, Allison had already missed thirty days of school. In November 1989, a psychological assessment (pre-injury) revealed average intellectual abilities, oppositional tendencies, immaturity and a poor self-image. It was recommended that she become involved in an outpatient day treatment program for drug/alcohol abusers, receive 1:1 counseling and that her family become involved with the counseling. Eight days prior to her injury, Allison was identified as an "adjudicated delinquent for accessory after the fact, theft in the second degree." Allison was a passenger in a car that was stolen. It was recommended that she be placed in her father's home.

Allison indicated that she was enthusiastic about participating in the follow-up evaluation as she felt it would help her get back into school. Findings during the evaluation included:
1) good general health, both Allison and father deny any current problems with alcohol.
2) sleeps for extended periods of time (sometimes sleeps as much as 12-14 hours/day)
3) occasional headaches
4) sometimes holds her head at an unusual angle when regarding objects or persons
5) flat affect throughout the day's evaluation; fatigued easily
6) neurological assessment clear
7) could not identify the day but knew the date; could not identify
the President of the United States
8) some decline noted on intellectual assessment; now (6 months post-injury)
functioning in the borderline range
9) problems with short term, episodic memory
10) mood swings
11) loss of sense of smell
12) trouble with written expression
13) expressed desire to return to school and indicated intentions to stay away from friends
with whom she had gotten into trouble in the past
14) academic skills within the sixth and seventh-grade with the exception of math, which was
at approximately a third grade level
15) exhibited rocking behavior throughout the day

Rehabilitation/Educational Team Recommendations:

1) enroll in summer school to work on cognitive/academic activities for a few hours each day; summer school will provide an opportunity for local education staff to observe her and identify an appropriate program for the fall

2) do not retain, primarily because of her age; provide individualized instruction where needed (particularly in math and written work)

3) light academic load at the beginning of the school year

4) provide and help supervise an "organization notebook" to assist with memory and organization

5) consider a buddy system to help with writing down assignments, moving from class to class, organizing locker and books, assisting with social interactions

6) involvement with local support group for family

7) place to lie down at school when she becomes fatigued

8) short school day if appropriate

9) case manager/school counselor to facilitate communication between all involved and to be available for Allison as needed; past history suggest that she will have difficulty with making responsible decisions

10) adapt for written work; peer secretary, keyboarding, reduce assignment length, oral completion of work

11) incorporate "life skills" in daily curriculum

12) increase structure, prompts and cues in all classes to ensure successful experiences

13) careful observation for symptoms that might suggest a seizure disorder

14) consider potential problems with visual field cuts

Follow-up evaluation approximately one year later revealed that Allison was now living with her mother and new stepfather; she reported "personality differences" with her father which precipitated the return to living with her mother. Allison's mother reported that Allison was "not as wild" and that she was less defiant at home. She described Allison as somewhat moody with a tendency to be impatient. Allison reported that she felt "left out" among her peers at school and commented that no one liked her. She also described herself as moody, occasionally depressed and nervous. Allison also presented numerous physical complaints including stomach aches, dizziness, swollen glands and constant fatigue. The local guidance counselor reported concern as Allison had indicated that she had been sexually active; he set up an appointment for her at a local family planning clinic. As of the follow up evaluation, Allison was still unable to attend more than half days at school because of excessive fatigue. It was recommended that further neurological workup be considered if Allison did not improve in terms of her stamina, energy level and sleep needs.

IV   Families and Educators: Creating Partnerships for Students with Brain Injuries

MARILYN LASH, M.S.W.

As children enter or return to school following a brain injury, parents expect that the worst is behind them. Few parents forget the horror of seeing their child injured and the fear that their child will not make it through the injury. Even years later, parents can still describe in painful detail their feelings of anguish and helplessness during the agonizing wait for news at the hospital. Seeing their child lying unresponsive and comatose is a living nightmare for parents that is only worsened by their guilt over failure to protect their child from harm.

Many parents spend long days and nights at the hospital while other children manage as best they can at home, often in the substitute care of relatives or neighbors. Children with more serious injuries are often transferred from local hospitals to trauma centers in urban areas for specialized care. This creates even more upheaval in the family's life. Living in motel rooms, sleeping in hospital waiting rooms, and taking turns at their child's bedside is physically and emotionally exhausting. Many parents hang on simply by holding on to the hope that if they can only get their child home, then everything will be all right.

A survey that was completed by 68 parents whose children had been injured seriously enough to be hospitalized in a pediatric trauma center or to be admitted to an inpatient rehabilitation program showed that they needed more information about the injury and its effects on their child. [1] The top four needs for information cited were: 1) the meaning of their child's diagnosis; 2) information about community organizations and resources; 3) availability of state and federal programs for children with disabilities; and 4) expectations for their child's future.

These needs underscore how unprepared families are for the physical, emotional, cognitive, and behavioral changes that may result from a brain injury. The grieving process that families experience is incomplete because the child makes it through the injury but is changed. The process is further complicated by the many unknown questions that physicians and other health care professionals are unable to answer. Little research has been done to study the long-term outcomes of children following brain injury.

The tendency of many children to make remarkable physical progress often masks more subtle changes in the child's ability to process information, organize tasks, control impulses, and monitor behaviors.

This uncertainty creates many conflicts and anxieties for families. The tendency of many children to make remarkable physical progress often masks more subtle changes in the child's ability to process information, organize tasks, control impulses, and monitor behaviors. For a child whose brain injury is considered less severe, and particularly a child who did not have the dramatic stage of coma, subtle changes in emotions, behaviors, and learning may puzzle families and educators. These difficulties usually become more apparent as the child enters or returns to school and is increasingly challenged to learn new information, adjust to multiple settings, interact with many students and teachers, and is expected to meet academic standards.

School is a critical environment for the child and family. It is the setting where children learn to function outside the shelter and protection of their homes and to develop the social skills necessary to develop and maintain interpersonal relationships. It is the arena where students gradually develop the skills and self-reliance that will enable them to become independent and to prepare them for adulthood. School is also the arena where the long-term and latent cognitive effects of a child's brain injury are most likely to become evident as the challenge of learning becomes increasingly complex.

The child who has had a brain injury is particularly at risk for lowered academic performance, social isolation, and lowered self-esteem. Depression is a common reaction among students with brain injuries who are aware of their inability to achieve pre-injury levels of academic performance and social integration. This failure is readily personalized into feelings of lowered self-worth that can lead to serious depression and withdrawal.

Educators are critical resources for interventions, guidance and support for students with brain injuries and for their parents. Educators can be the pivotal influence to prepare peers, develop support systems, identify needed interventions, design compensatory strategies, and develop academic and functional goals. It is important for educators to collaborate closely with parents or guardians throughout this process, yet too often the process of educational planning and negotiation for special education and related services becomes an adversarial one or occurs only after the student has had major difficulties or failures. The following section discusses primary concerns that have been identified by families for their child's return to school following a brain injury and during subsequent transitions in school between teachers, grades and schools.

Blame and guilt among families

Brain injuries among children most frequently result from motor vehicle related collisions. Children are injured by motor vehicles while riding as occupants, when struck as pedestrians, or involved in bicycling collisions. These mechanisms involve speed and impact. Falls from heights can also result in brain injuries among children. Common causes are falls down flights of stairs, out of windows, and off balconies.

Injuries are not isolated events. Not only may the child's brain be injured, but other body regions may be damaged as well. However, unlike bone fractures, cuts, bruises, and even internal injuries, brain injuries cause irreparable damage. The physical damage to a child is compounded by the emotional aftermath. Other persons - parents, siblings or peers - may be injured and hospitalized as well. Just at the time when a young child may most need the comfort and presence of a parent, they may be unavailable and separated. The death of a parent, sibling or peer can be devastating to the child who survives. The child who is hospitalized is even isolated from the mourning rituals of funerals. The full impact may not be felt until the child leaves the protective environment of the hospital and experiences the loss at home, in school, and in the community.

The tragedy of these injuries is that they can be prevented. Children wearing safety belts, placed in child safety seats, and wearing bicycle helmets are less likely to be seriously injured. Safety measures such as protective rails and guards can protect children from falls. Parents experience terrible anguish and guilt over their failure to protect their child from harm as they relive "if only I had" scenarios.

A child's injury affects every member of the family in some way. The grieving and adjustment process for families is described in the guide "When your child is seriously injured....the emotional impact on families." Based on the input and experiences of families, it traces the reactions of families from arrival at the emergency room through the child's hospitalization and planning for discharge. It is recommended to give educators insight into the emotional trauma that families experience, including siblings, and contains many practical suggestions for coping.

Educators are critical resources for interventions, guidance and support for students with brain injuries and for their parents.

The process of a family's grieving is unpredictable. Marital stress is common when spouses cope in different ways. Some parents recall feeling so totally overwhelmed that they isolated themselves at home, cried constantly and avoided friends and neighbors. Others coped by becoming extremely busy and involved. As friends or teachers admired how well they were doing, they were terrified of falling apart if they stopped. In their grief, families may seek someone to blame, to become the target of their anger. It is possible for schools or teachers to become this target just as a physician or nurse was at the hospital. It is important to understand that the anger may stem from a deeper grief and rage about what has happened to the child.

Denial is a term used to describe the feeling that, "It can't be true, it's not real, it can't be as bad as they say." Professionals in health care and educators often view denial as a negative symptom and become frustrated with parents because they "aren't facing the facts." Denial is actually a protective stage that can help families function as they gather the emotional strength to deal with their losses.

The word "acceptance" is often used, but is a difficult and lengthy process. How long it takes to reach this stage is different for each parent. One way of describing it is the point at which parents have a realistic understanding of their child's abilities and limitations. It is that period when the child with the injury's condition and care are no longer the central focus in a family's life. While the child may always have special needs, they do not necessarily take priority over the needs of others in the family, but are balanced within the needs of all for care, attention, support and love.

What is rehabilitation?

A child's recovery from a brain injury is not limited to a specific time period or place of treatment. Discharge from an acute hospital or rehabilitation program does not signal a child's recovery from a brain injury. Rather, discharge from the hospital marks the beginning of the next stage of rehabilitation that will occur in the child's home and school. Rehabilitation is a long-term process that will continue throughout the child's development and has no defined end point.

Rehabilitation services are very different for children than for adults. There are not many pediatric rehabilitation programs specializing in brain injury. According to the National Pediatric Trauma Registry, more children with four or more functional limitations are discharged directly home from trauma centers than are transferred to in-patient rehabilitation programs. The leading diagnosis among these children is brain injury.

Another contributing factor is the family's ability to provide physical care at home despite difficulties in mobility, dressing, bathing, speech, vision, hearing, cognition or behavior. Children are lighter and smaller; this enables families to provide care at home that would otherwise be impossible for adults. Still another factor is the limits of health insurance benefits for children. Many policies do not cover in-patient rehabilitation services; thus, limiting options for families.

Consequently, educators will encounter children with brain injuries who spend many weeks or months in rehabilitation hospitals and programs before returning home. However, they will also meet children who return directly home from the acute care hospital or trauma center. Length of stay in a hospital does not determine whether a child will need special education after a brain injury. In fact, the family whose child has returned directly home after a short hospital stay may be even less prepared to assess the long-term consequences of their child's injury and be less prepared to discuss educational needs with the school.

...discharge from the hospital marks the beginning of the next stage of rehabilitation that will occur in the child's home and school.

Families lack prior experience with special education

The vast majority of children who have brain injuries have no preexisting conditions. Consequently, their parents are inexperienced with the "special needs" system and may consider it a program primarily for children with birth disorders or mental retardation.

The primary question that families ask is, "How will my child's brain injury affect his/her ability to learn?" Unfortunately, medical and rehabilitation experts can not give parents precise or definitive information. Although P.L. 101-476, the Individuals with Disabilities Education Act, specifically creates a special classification for children with traumatic brain injuries, the provision of services still needs to be negotiated individually with the child's local school and educational systems. Families need basic information about:

- What is special education?
- How do I apply for my child?
- What does my child need?
- How do I know if I can trust this teacher?
- How can I tell if my child is learning?
- How can I measure my child's progress?

Family's concerns about qualifications of educators

Families often refer to discharge from the hospital or rehabilitation program as the second "crisis of injury" because the responsibility for the child's ongoing care and continuing needs shifts to them. During the medical crisis, families draw reassurance from the multiple specialists caring for their child. Knowing that their child is "in the hands of experts" brings some comfort. By contrast when the child returns to school, families typically find that educators and school staff have little or no prior experience or training in brain injury. This creates considerable anxiety and even alarm. How will the school know what my child needs?

Unfortunately, this contrast is often reinforced by recommendations from medical and rehabilitation experts that specialized services and programs in brain injury are needed for the child at school. Recommendations may be made for a specialized classroom, expensive testing, and special programming that is unavailable at the local school. Families are ill prepared to judge whether alternative methods of instruction and services proposed by the school are adequate.

The time required by schools to gather medical information, complete testing, apply for services, and construct educational plans often takes much longer than families expect. It contrasts with the rapid pace of the child's earlier medical treatment. Meanwhile, many parents become anxious about the effects of these delays upon their child's progress and recovery.

Educators can build confidence in parents by showing an interest and willingness to learn about the effects of brain injuries. Parents stressed that it is the interest, flexibility and commitment by teachers that fostered positive relationships. While parents would have preferred that teachers already have specialized skills and training in brain injuries, many recognize the limitations of schools and teachers' experiences. When teachers were receptive to suggestions for reading and to information from state brain injury chapters, as well as the idea of being available for consultation with rehabilitation staff, inquired about strategies used by parents, and asked insightful questions, then parents were reassured and felt that their child was less "at risk" in school.

Timing of child's return to school

The length of a child's hospitalization is not a predictor of what the child will need upon returning to school. The severity of the injury is not the same as the severity of the disability that may result. Some children with very serious injuries recover quite well. Others with less severe brain injuries have long lasting difficulties. The length of time that a child is absent following an injury can affect how educators and families perceive the child's needs. When a child is in critical condition, particularly when a coma extends for weeks or months, schools are alerted to the possibility that this child may have a serious disability. The child who is seen briefly in the emergency room and sent home, or admitted overnight for observation after a blow to the head is more readily assumed to be "all right." This is not always true.

Each brain injury is different. Any child whose behaviors and performance at school changes following a blow to the head should raise questions about whether the brain has been injured.

The transfer of information between medical specialists and educators frequently is problematic. School staff often assume that the medical staff will advise them of what is needed, while medical staff wait for the school to contact them. Too often, the result is poor communication and preplanning between hospitals and schools. When schools do receive medical reports, they are frequently written in such technical medical jargon that they are of little use for educational planning.

As a last resort, families become the link for information between hospital staff, follow-up appointments and school staff. However, families may not know what information is needed, how to collect it, and what to do with it. A detailed outline of the physical, sensory, communicative, cognitive and behavioral effects of brain injuries was developed for families in the guide, "When your child goes to school after an injury." It lists questions for families to ask educators about their child's abilities and performance at school. Educators may wish to use this as a guide.

Medical and educational institutions are completely different entities in terms of how they are staffed, financed and operated. These fundamental differences can lead to conflicts in expectations and goals as the child with brain injury moves from one setting to the other.

Miracle of recovery

Families frequently describe their child's recovery from a life threatening injury as miraculous. Having seen their child close to death, in a coma, breathing only with the help of a respirator, wired to machines and hooked into tubes, is a terrifying experience. Even when a child slowly emerges from coma, many families are given cautious predictions about the child's functional abilities for mobility, speech, communication, and self-care. Having watched a child beat the grim odds given by medical experts, it is not surprising that many parents expect the same miraculous recovery to extend into school.

This "need to hope" is also a reflection of how weary and exhausted families can be by the time a child is ready to return to school. Going to school may signal a respite for families from the child's daily care and supervision, from the stress of lowered finances due to time off from work and unpaid medical bills. Consequently, families may be unprepared to face the difficulties that their child may experience in school. If the school adopts an attitude of "Let's wait and see" how the child does in school, the family may be only too willing to "hope for the best" because they are exhausted. However, this delay can result in lost opportunities for early intervention for educational planning

The child who is seen briefly in the emergency room and sent home, or admitted overnight for observation after a blow to the head is more readily assumed to be "all right." This is not always true.

and the student may be quickly discouraged by early failures and difficulty adjusting to the demands of the classroom and curriculum.

Families need careful and supportive guidance by school staff to make sure that the child's needs are thoroughly assessed and that educational plans are designed as soon as possible to address the child's special learning needs. The initial "honeymoon period" between schools and families often ceases when it becomes evident that the child is encountering serious difficulties. Too often, negotiations deteriorate into legal battles between schools and families. The following suggestions are designed to prevent this from occurring and to encourage a partnership for educational planning between parents and educators.

Parents can detect subtle changes before they are apparent to others.

■ Listen to families

Parents know their child best. They not only have the pre-injury comparison of how their child is functioning, but they have seen their child's reactions and progress through the various stages of treatment and recovery. Parents can detect subtle changes before they are apparent to others. This is particularly important with younger children who are unable to express their needs clearly. Families also have opportunities to observe their child's cognitive process in many different settings and circumstances. Parents see how their child functions during days and evenings, when tired or alert, in concentrated silence or with distracting interruptions. Parents and family members have experience in developing cueing systems, in designing strategies to aid memory, and helping children finish tasks. Parents' observations may yield information that is far more practical than testing and achievement scores that represent the child's capacity in a structured and controlled setting for specific functions.

Carryover and consistency between families and educators is essential for the child who has had a brain injury. Therefore, it is important for educators and families to share their methods so that the family can reinforce effective techniques used in the classroom. Similarly, educators may find home based strategies that parents have found effective to be applicable with modifications to the classroom setting.

■ Set up a record keeping system with families

Many children return for follow-up visits to medical specialists long after their injuries yet reports are frequently not shared with schools. The family is the critical link and can facilitate communication by requesting copies of reports and delivering them directly. A child's recovery is likely to extend over years. During this time families will meet with many specialists, educators, and consultants. Children will have many assessments done, testing performed, reports written and recommendations made. None of this information is likely to be stored in one place and can be just about impossible to track down years later. As children progress through grades and various schools, bits and pieces inevitably get lost or separated.

Families and educators can benefit right in the beginning by setting up an educational record in a flexible three ring binder that remains the property of the parent. This record will grow as the child moves from teacher to teacher, grade to grade and school to school. Educators and families can strategize what information is most useful to record. This can provide a critical and comprehensive record that can be used by families and educators to track a child's progress, to compare interventions and program results, to record important dates, names and addresses. It provides a continuous record that can be useful to identify patterns, spot potential problems and compare programs and results.

Suggestions for sections to include are:

■ Description of pre-injury history in school

■ Description of medical care and rehabilitation

■ Community resources

■ State and federal programs

■ Description of major abilities and difficulties for child

■ Past and current academic grades and performance

■ Special education directors, teachers, teacher aids, and tutors

■ Special education services recommended and received

■ Related services such as transportation, therapies, counseling, etc.

■ Altering hopes and dreams

Uncertainty about the future is one of the most difficult aspects of brain injury for families. The loss of hopes and dreams is painful. The age when the child is injured is a factor. Parents of children who were very young when injured speak of the lost potential. When preschool age children are injured, or even very young elementary school children, so much is still unknown about the child's skills, abilities and interests. The child's personality is still emerging as communication skills develop, as habits form and unique character traits appear. Parents speak wistfully of not knowing how their child "might have been" had the injury not occurred.

A particular sadness expressed by parents of children injured during their earlier formative years is the sadness of watching younger siblings surpass them in motor skills, communication and speech, and cognitive abilities. Siblings of children injured at a young age also quickly lose their recall of the child prior to injury. The competition that parents must tolerate but expect between siblings has a bittersweet edge after an injury when the younger siblings' abilities surpass the older child who has been injured.

When an adolescent child is injured, aspirations for jobs, vocational training careers, and college already may be defined. A brain injury may seriously threaten these plans and force families, students and educators to reevaluate whether they are realistic. Peer pressures among adolescents can make it especially difficult for the student who has had a brain injury to fit in and keep up with classmates. Appearance, dating, and sexuality become primary concerns among adolescents and the injured student may no longer be as attractive to and accepted by peers.

> **Peer pressures among adolescents can make it especially difficult for the student who has had a brain injury to fit in and keep up with classmates.**

Too many high school students who were injured close to graduation have accepted high school diplomas without realizing that they have disqualified themselves for additional special educational services. This premature graduation can readily backfire as students find that vocational rehabilitation services in the community are not as readily available as education in public schools. Any family with an adolescent approaching graduation age needs careful advice and guidance from educators on whether acceptance of a diploma effects eligibility for further educational services and vocational options. A transition plan that identifies how the student will acquire the necessary skills for adulthood is needed.

■ Foster families

Child abuse is a primary cause of brain injury among infants and preschool children. Foster and adoptive families typically lack complete medical records and family histories for these children. Many abused children have multiple disabilities including damaged vision or hearing as well as motor difficulties. Multiple foster homes and temporary placements can contribute to behavioral problems and exacerbate emotional disturbances among abused children. This can contribute to delinquent patterns and even expulsion from school. The significance of early brain injuries caused by beatings or batterings may be overlooked as the child ages. Because children's brains are especially vulnerable to injury if abused or beaten at an early age, it is important for foster families and educators to question the relationship between early physical abuse and learning difficulties and behaviors.

■ Do not forget siblings

Brothers and sisters are often the forgotten people in cases of brain injuries. With the primary concern and attention directed at the child who is brain injured, siblings can easily be overlooked. The turmoil at home inevitably affects siblings. Young siblings may mistakenly believe they are somehow to blame for the injury as the young child's thinking often confuses cause and effect. Siblings may have witnessed the injury and have recurrent nightmares, fears, or trouble sleeping. Siblings may be jealous at the attention focused on the child with brain injury and resent the disruptions in the family's routine. Older siblings may have additional responsibilities of caring for others and managing the household while parents are at the hospital.

These stresses may become evident at school as the grades of siblings drop, as attention wanders, or as behaviors change. Families may fail to inform the teachers of siblings about the family crisis. Consequently, as schools are advised of a child's injury, they should inform the teachers of siblings. School staff can then be alert to changes in siblings' behavior and grades and provide additional attention, support, and counseling.

Additional Information

The following materials are available from the Research and Training Center in rehabilitation and Childhood Trauma and can be requested by contacting: 750 Washington St, #75K-R, Boston, MA 02111 (tel. 617-956-5032).

When your child is seriously injured: The emotional impact on families
When your child goes to school after an injury
Rehab Update - 12 page newsletter
National Pediatric Trauma Registry Information Packet
Strategies for Educators: A Packet for schools and families
Publications Catalog on Rehabilitation of Childhood Trauma

The author grants permission to reprint this chapter either in part or in its entirety.

1   *Communication between Parents and Professionals cited as Top Need. Rehab Update, Research and Training Center on Rehabilitation and Childhood Trauma, Summer, 1993*

V Educational Assessment of Students with Brain Injuries

JOAN CARNEY, ED.D.

Focus:

Educational Assessment as Part of the Interdisciplinary Evaluation Process

Domains Requiring Investigation

Physical Factors Affecting Evaluation

Interpretation of Results

The nature of brain injury, its sudden onset, and its impact on all aspects of behavior necessitate that the educator alter many of his/her traditional practices in educational assessment. When to evaluate, what areas to explore, the physical adaptations that may be necessary, as well as the differences in how to interpret results all have an impact on this process. In these cases the educator's task is not to diagnose, as they know brain injury has occurred. In order to design an educational program the educator needs to assess a variety of cognitive functions for presence and degree of impairment. Much research to date has established that these cognitive and psychosocial sequelae of brain injury are considered more debilitating than resulting motoric deficits. Interpretation, then, must be made within the context of research and clinical experience with children with brain injury.

Professionals should guard against repeating specific instruments but, it is these multiple opportunities to observe behaviors that lend the insight needed to plan an effective educational program.

Interdisciplinary Evaluation

Federal legislation designed to protect the rights of children has lead educational professionals to adopt a set of widely used practices. Among them is the requirement for a "multidisciplinary" evaluation. When learning problems are suspected, psychological and educational assessments are arranged with assessments in related services areas recommended on only a case by case basis. Especially when evaluating a child with brain injury, all areas of cognitive, social/behavioral, and sensorimotor function should be assessed. Hence, the need for an interdisciplinary model so that various professionals can coordinate and merge their diagnostic findings.

Optimally, the members of the assessment team have had experience treating, teaching, and counseling children with acquired brain injury. Such children exhibit both obvious and more subtle changes in each aspect of their behavior that can be best interpreted and remediated by experienced practitioners. It is unlikely that a local educational agency will be able to offer such experience due to the relatively small percentages of children with brain injury in each locality. Some well informed educational systems are exploring the option of identifying a regional team of professionals who can provide the necessary assessments, or consult with local practitioners regarding their findings. Where such a team is not in place, families and local educational agencies can look to rehabilitative treatment centers and private agencies for such specialized experience.

In any interdisciplinary evaluation there is, and should be, an overlap of areas assessed. For example, the psychological or neuropsychological assessment, along with its primary purpose, will generally screen such areas as academic achievement. The educator will assess academic mastery thoroughly and only screen those processing modalities that will be more carefully evaluated by other disciplines. Perceptual and sensorimotor function will likely be investigated by the neuropsychologist, the occupational therapist and the educator in their evaluations. Professionals should guard against repeating specific instruments but, it is these multiple opportunities to observe behaviors that lend the insight needed to plan an effective educational program. These various perspectives of a deficit area can help to predict a child's performance in educational and social settings.

In a rehabilitative setting, ongoing screenings are necessary for adjustments to treatment as the patient changes during the dynamic neurologic recovery phase. Medical professionals will rarely predict the degree of recovery for a child who has sustained brain injury; the majority will, however, continue to look for some degree of continued neurologic recovery over several years. Those assessing a student in order to design an educational program following brain injury should not necessarily await the end of spontaneous recovery. Medical stability and a slowing in the pace of recovery will mark the appropriate time for the multidisciplinary evaluation and subsequent return to an appropriate educational program. At this point, the student should be oriented to time, place and event and they should possess the ability to sustain attention for approximately thirty minutes at a time.

Once an educational program is in place, traditional practices call for review in sixty days and then yearly. A child who has sustained a brain injury needs to be evaluated formally and informally on an ongoing basis to monitor their continued spontaneous recovery and to evaluate the compensations and adaptations made for reintegration to a school program. For the first year, this should take place every thirty to sixty days. In subsequent years the frequency of the review process may slow as dictated by the student's continued rate of change.

Educational Assesment

The educational portion of an interdisciplinary evaluation typically measures academic achievement, learning style, and school performance in comparison to a local or national norm group. Here we are presented with several problems when considering the child with brain injury. First, those cognitive and behavioral sequelae of brain injury which will likely affect school performance may not be investigated in a traditional educational battery. Second, sensorimotor impairments following brain injury are likely to impact upon the choice and administration of assessment instruments. Third, comparison to norm groups is not the only, or best, comparison to be made and lastly, academic achievement levels at this point in time do not reflect or predict the potential for new learning of a student who has sustained a brain injury.

Areas of Investigation

Any aspect of behavior may be affected by brain injury in one of at least three ways: loss of function, decrease in function, or increase in function. The interdisciplinary evaluation team must rely on each member to focus on these changes in their respective areas but, those most prevalent sequelae of brain injury should be assessed by all disciplines. Discussed in earlier chapters as cognitive, social/behavioral, and sensorimotor disorders, the following represent more specific areas affected in many children who have sustained brain injury:

■ **communication and language**
■ **any or all types of perception**
■ **attention and concentration**
■ **judgment and reasoning**
■ **self-esteem and self-awareness**
■ **motivation and initiation**
■ **appropriate social behavior**
■ **sensory input**
■ **speed and coordination of movement**
■ **speed of processing input and output**
■ **motor function**
■ **speech**
■ **any or all types of memory**

In his/her assessment, the educator must look at academic achievement, potential for new learning, and orientation to educational and noneducational tasks that typically occur in a school environment. The following table lists suggested areas of investigation in the educational assessment as well as some instruments which may be helpful in assessing function in that domain. Some of the tests listed have training and credentials restrictions but most are available for use by educators without supervision. This table is by no means exhaustive and represents suggested instruments to be administered after careful selection of a battery appropriate to the developmental level and physical characteristics of the child in question. In general, academic functioning should be fully assessed and each of the other areas screened for their effect on functioning in a school setting. Under no circumstances should a student be administered all of these tests and there must be communication among the members of the interdisciplinary evaluation team to prevent repetition of a particular instrument.

Areas of Investigation	Suggested Instrument
Academic Functioning	Woodcock-Johnson Psycho-Educational Battery-Revised (WJPEB-R), standard and supplemental achievement subtests
	Kaufman Test of Educational Achievement (KTEA)
	Peabody Individual Achievement Tests-Revised (PIAT-R)
	Gates-MacGinitie Reading Tests
	Key Math-Revised
	Informal Reading Inventory
	School Function Assessment
	Test of Written Language-2 (TOWL-2)
	Test of Early Reading Ability-2 (TERA-2)
	Test of Early Mathematics Ability (TEMA-2)
Attention and Concentration	Detroit Tests of Learning Aptitude-Primary (DTLA-P)
	WJPEB-R Cognitive Abilities, Memory for Names, Memory for Sentences, Visual-Auditory Learning, Memory for Words, Cross Out, Visual Matching
	Detroit Tests of Learning Aptitude-2 (DTLA-2), Sentence Imitation, Oral Directions, Word Sequences, Design Reproduction, Object Sequences, Letter Sequences
	Seashore Rhythm Test
	Corsi Block Tapping Test

Areas of Investigation	Suggested Instrument
Attention and Concentration (con.)	Matching Familiar Figures Test
	Continuous Performance Test
	Trail Making Tests
	Paced Auditory Serial Addition Test
Memory/New Learning	DTLA-P
	DTLA-2, Sentence Imitation, Oral Directions, Word Sequences, Design Reproduction, Object Sequences, Letter Sequences
	Kaufmann Assessment Battery for Children (KABC)
	WJPEB-R Cognitive Abilities, Memory for Names, Memory for Sentences, Visual-Auditory Learning, Memory for Words
	Rey-Osterrieth Complex Figure Recall
	Selective Reminding Test
	California Verbal Learning Test
	Learning Efficiency Test
	Revised Visual Retention Test
	Test of Visual Perceptual Skills (TVPS)
Reasoning	WJPEB-R Cognitive Abilities, Analysis-Synthesis, Concept Formation
	Test of Nonverbal Intelligence (TONI)
	Differential Aptitude Tests
	DTLA-2, Word Opposites, Story Construction, Symbolic Relations, Conceptual Matching, Word Fragments
	Ross Test of Higher Cognitive Processes

Areas of Investigation	Suggested Instrument
Communication/Language Processing	TOWL-2
	DTLA-2, Word Opposites, Sentence Imitation, Oral Directions, Word Sequences, Story Construction, Word Fragments, Conceptual Matching
	DTLA-P
	Revised Token Test
	WJPEB-R Cognitive Abilities, Memory for Sentences, Incomplete Words, Picture Vocabulary, Oral Vocabulary, Listening Comprehension, Verbal Analogies, Sound Blending, Sound Patterns
	Peabody Picture Vocabulary Test (PPVT)
	Expressive One Word Picture Vocabulary Test (EOWPVT)
	Informal Reading Inventory, Hearing Capacity subtest
	Test of Early Language Development (TELD)
Visual Perception/Visual-Motor Integration/ Reproduction, Object Sequences, Letter Sequences, Symbolic Relations, Word Fragments	DTLA-2, Oral Directions, Design Processing Speed
	DTLA-P
	WJPEB-R Cognitive Abilities, Visual Matching, Visual Closure, Picture Recognition, Spatial Relations, Cross Out
	Developmental Test of Visual-Motor Integration
	TVPS
	Bender Gestalt Test for Children
	Rey-Osterrieth Complex Figure Drawing
	TONI

Areas of Investigation	Suggested Instrument
Socioemotional Adjustment	Child Behavior Checklist, Parent and Teacher Report Forms (pre- and post-traumatically) Conners Checklist Cognitive Behavior Rating Scales

Executive functioning is often affected by brain injury because such injuries frequently involve the frontal lobes. Thus, executive functions such as volition, self-awareness, planning, making choices, self-regulation, and self- monitoring are often disturbed. Formal testing, by its nature, compensates for many of brain injuries' debilitating executive impairments. To assess a student who has sustained brain injury regarding their potential for new learning and orientation to the educational environment, educators must add naturalistic assessments to their standardized batteries. Traits such as goal setting, planning, independent direction, motivation, and initiation are typically overlooked in assessment and the interpretation of findings yet, they are necessary for success in most educational settings.

Two means of investigating such areas are through observation and interview. Observations, though they are ecologic, should not be random. Facets which should be systematically considered in an observation are the parameters of the task, environmental factors, the guidelines for measuring the quality or quantity of the behaviors, and the degree of cues and compensation used to complete the task. Because many functions are subject to disruption, many samples of behavior should be considered. Interview of a family member or primary therapist will more closely report the student's function in a natural environment and usually identify problems not noted in formal testing. Some areas to inquire about in an interview might be: attention length and quality; flexibility in shifting tasks; use of compensatory strategies; insight into deficits; new learning ability; response to stress; initiation; and judgment and problem solving. Information obtained by observation and interview may also lead the educator to choose a formal instrument in an attempt to more clearly define or quantify a deficit area.

> Some areas to inquire about in an interview might be: attention length and quality; flexibility in shifting tasks; use of compensatory strategies; insight into deficits; new learning ability; response to stress; initiation; and judgment and problem solving.

Physical Factors

Many physical factors need to be considered in the selection and administration of test instruments for the child who has sustained a brain injury. The most obvious among them is stamina. Fatigue and headaches are common physical symptoms following brain injury and should be considered not only when making plans for school reintegration, but during the evaluation process as well. Administration of the educational assessment should be broken down into several sessions, with length being dictated by the student's needs. Interdisciplinary assessment team members should also coordinate their evaluation sessions so as not to overwhelm the child. In some cases, evaluations in more physically active disciplines such as occupational and physical therapy can be interspersed with more sedentary ones to provide variety for the child.

Ability to gain, sustain, and shift attention must also be considered in assessing the student who has a brain injury. Although information about a child's attention span will be important to planning educational intervention, varying the tasks within each evaluation session may prove necessary or helpful when assessing the student with attentional difficulties as a result of brain injury.

Brain injury can cause physical disorders effecting access to information (input) and available response modes (output). For example, cortical blindness or visual field defects are not uncommon in children who have sustained severe brain injury. This clearly puts limits on instrument selection and may dictate the positioning or size of visual stimuli presented. Hearing deficits seem to be less prominent but, many children who have sustained brain injury complain of difficulty in hearing. For some children, this is later determined to be a problem of auditory processing (memory, comprehension, aphasia, or attention). Regardless, this sensory disturbance will also require careful consideration in the selection of instruments and in the interpretation of their results.

Impulsivity and distractibility are also common following brain injury.

Impulsivity and distractibility are also common following brain injury. Although formal test manuals usually address the testing environment, these recommendations for a quiet, distraction-free setting should be taken seriously especially in the case of the child with acquired brain injury. If the educator wishes to gather further data on a student's tendency toward impulsivity and distractibility, they may plan to observe them across several settings.

Motoric impairment can also pose difficulties in response mode for the child with brain injury. For example, dysarthric speech may alter subtest selection to those requiring pointing rather than verbal responses. Otherwise, the examiner may choose to allow the subject to respond in writing. Similarly, upper extremity motoric deficits may prohibit a student from providing a written response and thus keyboard access may be necessary or written language may be left unassessed. The examiner should first attempt to choose subtests which can be administered as they were standardized. Any alterations in standard procedures must be described in the examiner's written report and scores should be interpreted cautiously but, much information regarding a student's approach to a task and functioning in an academic setting can be obtained from allowing these adaptations.

Another technique that can be employed in some situations serves not only to adjust for some of these difficulties but also to quantify their impact. It is a system of double scoring. For example, the examiner may score an error for standard presentation and response and then readminister the item providing the student with rewording or simplification of the stimuli presented, scoring this subsequent response as well. The optimized score can then be compared to the standard one for discrepancy and also serves as a measure of the student's potential when provided such remediation. The provision of verbal cues, visual prompts, direct instruction, and modeling by the examiner can supply the basis for program recommendations and optimal methods of instruction.

Comparison of Performance

Although comparison to a norm group gives us some insight into how a student might perform in an age appropriate setting, more importantly in the case of brain injury, is how the child's performance compares with pre-injury levels. Comparing a student with himself, pre- and post-injury, should best inform educational professionals of those necessary adaptations to be made within regular or special education programming. Test scores and observations that describe a student's behavior as within normal limits may not appear to be problematic. However, study habits developed prior to brain injury may not be adequate post-traumatically and the student will become subject to unexplained failure. Any alteration in functioning needs to be identified and compensated for in educational plans.

Prior school records are an excellent source of pre-traumatic data. Most school-aged youngsters are routinely given standardized achievement batteries yielding comparisons with age or grade peers. Students with previous exceptionalities may also have individualized intelligence or achievement data available in their educational record. This information should be carefully considered as it provides an effective frame of reference.

As other neurobehavioral factors have a greater impact on educational performance following brain injury, it is vital to acquire pre- and post-traumatic behavioral inventories. These interviews are subjective by nature and in such an emotionally charged situation, many youngsters tend to be remembered only at their best. This factor makes it advisable to obtain such pre-traumatic data as soon as possible from a variety of informants. Family members and previous teachers should be interviewed, or asked to complete formal surveys as soon as possible following the onset of brain injury.

Interpretation of Findings

Academic achievement tests measure achieved mastery or prior learning. In most students, the rate of learning to date allows an evaluator to predict the student's continued rate of mastery. Such is not true in the case of the child who has sustained a brain injury. Fortunately, for these children, much academic mastery is so overlearned that it remains intact following brain injury. Skills in the encoding and decoding of language, as well as the following of mathematics processes and the knowledge of science and social studies facts are important, but less so if they cannot be utilized effectively to acquire new learning. Thus, scores that place students within normal limits in academic achievement are only valuable in identifying appropriate units of study. Methods of instruction, necessary compensatory strategies, adaptations to the environment and behavioral strategies must be determined by the results of a variety of other subtests, interviews, and clinical observations.

> For example, poor performance on a verbal reasoning task may be due to word retrieval difficulties rather than verbal reasoning.

Subtests such as those suggested in the table provided in this chapter are meant to assess a variety of areas important to new learning. Scores cannot be interpreted without close clinical assessment of their meaning. For example, poor performance on a verbal reasoning task may be due to word retrieval difficulties rather than verbal reasoning. Low scores on a multiple choice test of reading or mathematics may be due to an undiagnosed visual field deficit prohibiting the student from viewing all of the various choices. Subtests designed to assess memory or many other executive functions may yield poor results due to the child's inability to sustain attention or their tendency toward impulsivity. Though all of these results are valuable in the overall assessment, the educator must be careful to report findings in light of the many factors which may enter into assessment of the child with brain injury.

Another prevalent sequela of brain injury is reduced efficiency in many cognitive and sensorimotor functions. Administering both timed and untimed subtests will assist in quantifying that which the examiner has observed clinically. In designing educational programs it is also crucial to consider not only academic skills but efficiency in meeting the often rigorous demands of our traditional educational system. For example, a student who has sustained brain injury may appear to have made a full recovery. Such children, when they return to school without proper evaluation, frequently meet with unexplained difficulty that is easily misinterpreted as a lack of motivation or a behavioral problem but, is in reality an inefficiency related to the organic brain damage.

In interpreting the findings of their educational assessment for these children, the educator must consider the impact of the injury on all aspects of a student's behavior. Teachers need to consider the factors stemming from its sudden and late onset and they must assess areas of importance to both academic and nonacademic school functioning. Each score and observation should be analyzed in light of what it purports to measure but should also be task-analyzed to examine whether the difficulty lies in a component or precursor skill. It is important to keep in mind the broad range of sequelae that may exist as a result of brain injury and the unique set of strengths and needs that each student who has sustained a brain injury is likely to manifest.

References

Achenbach, T. M., and Edelbrock, C.S. (1986a). Child Behavior Checklist and Youth Self-report. Burlington, VT: Author.

Achenbach, T.M. and Edelbrock, C.S. (1986b). Teachers Report Form. Burlington, VT: Author.

Beery, K. E. (1989). Developmental test of visual-motor integration. Cleveland, OH: Modern Curriculum Press.

Begali, V. (1987) . Head Injury in Children and Adolescents. Brandon, VT: Clinical Psychology Publishing Company.

Bennet, G., Seashore, N. , and Wesman, A.G. (1982). Differential aptitude tests. New York: The Psychological Corporation, Harcourt Brace Jovanovich Publishers.

Benton, A.L. (1974). The revised visual retention test. New York: Psychological Corporation.

Brown, L., Sherbenou, R.J., and Johnson, S.K. (1982). The test of nonverbal intelligence. Austin, TX: Pro-Ed Publishers.

Conners, C.K. (1985). The Conners Rating Scales: Instruments for the Assessment of Childhood Psychopathology. Unpublished manuscript, Childrens Hospital National Medical Center, Washington, DC.

Connolly, A.J., Nachtman, W. and Pritchett, E.M. (1988). Key math revised. Circle Pines, MN:American Guidance Service.

Delis, D.C., Kramer, J., Kaplan, E. and Ober, B.A. (1986). The California verbal learning test. San Antonio, TX:Psychological Corporation.

DiSimoni, F.G. (1978). Token Test for Children. Allen, TX: DLM Teaching Resources.

Dunn, L.M. and Dunn, L.M. (1981). Peabody picture vocabulary test revised. Circle Pines, MN: American Guidance Service.

Fay, G. and Janesheski, J. (1986). Neuropsychological assessment of head injured children. Journal of Head Trauma Rehabilitation, 1986;1(4): 16-21.

Gardner, M.F. (1979). Expressive one-word picture vocabulary test. Novato, CA: Academic Therapy Publications.

Gardner, M.F. (1982).Test of visual-perceptual skills (non motor). Seattle, WA: Special Child Publications.

Ginsburg, H. P. and Baroody, A. J. (1989). Test of early mathematics ability-2. Austin, TX: Pro-Ed Publishers.

Gronwall, D.M. (1977). A paced auditory serial addition task: A measure of recovery from concussion. Perceptual and Motor Skills, 44, 367-373.

Hammill, D.D. (1985). Detroit tests of learning aptitude (dtla-2). Austin, TX: Pro-Ed Publishers.

Hammill, D.D., and Larsen, S.C. (1983). Test of written language. Austin, TX: Pro-Ed Publishers.

Hresko, W. P., Reid, D.K., and Hammill, D.D. (1981). The test of early language development. Austin, TX: Pro-Ed Publishers.

Kaufman, A.S., and Kaufman, N. L. (1985). Kaufman test of educational achievement. Circle Pines, MN: American Guidance Service.

Koppitz, E. M., (1975). The Bender gestalt test for young children. New York, NY: Grune and Stratton Inc.

MacGinitie, W. H., and MacGinitie, R.K. (1989). Gates MacGinitie reading tests. Chicago, IL: Riverside Publishing.

Mack, J. (1986). Clinical assessment of disorders of attention and memory. Journal of Head Trauma Rehabilitation 1986; 1(3): 22-33.

Markwardt, F. C. (1989). Peabody individual achievement test-revised. Circle Pines, MN: American Guidance Service.

McNeill, M.R., and Prescott, T.E. (1978). Revised token test. Baltimore, MD: University Park Press.27. Milner, B. (1971). Interhemispheric differences in the localization of psychological processes in man. British Medical Bulletin, 27, 272-277.

Reid, D. K., Hresko, W. P., and Hammill, D.D. (1989). Test of early reading ability-2. Austin, TX: Pro-Ed Publishers.

Reitan, H.M. (1969). Manual for the administration of neuropsychological test batteries for adults and children. Tuscon, AZ: Neuropsychology Laboratory.

Reitan, R.M. and Davison, L.A. (1974). Clinical Neuropsychology: Current Status and Applications. Washington, DC: V.H. Winston.

Ross, D.G. (1986). Ross Information Processing Assessment. Austin, TX: Pro-Ed Publishers.

Ruff, R., Levin, H. and Marshall, L. (1986). Neurobehavioral methods of assessment and the study of outcome in minor head injury. Journal of Head Trauma Rehabilitation 1986;1(2): 43-52.

Savage, R. and Wolcott, G. (Eds) (1988). Educational Dimensions of Acquired Brain Injury. Austin, TX: Pro-Ed Publishers.

Silvaroli, N.J. (1986). Classroom Reading Inventory (5th ed.). Dubuque, IA: Wm. C. Brown.

Sohlberg, M. and Mateer, C. (1989). The assessment of cognitive-communicative functions in head injury. Topics in Language Disorders, 1989; 9(2): 15-33.

Waaland, P. (1990). Practical applications of child clinical neuropsychology. Presented at Cognitive Rehabilitation and Community Reintegration, Richmond, VA. September 13, 1990.

Webster, R.E., (1981). Learning efficiency test. Noveto, CA: Academic Therapy Publications.

Williams, J.M. (1987). Cognitive behavior rating Scales. Odessa, FL: Psychological Assessment Resources.

Wilson, B. and Moffat, N.(Eds) (1984). Clinical Management of Memory Problems. Rockville, MD: Aspen Publishers, Inc.ehavior rating Scales. Odessa, FL: Psychological Assessment Resources.

Wilson, B. and Moffat, N.(Eds) (1984). Clinical Management of Memory Problems. Rockville, MD: Aspen Publishers, Inc.

Woodcock, R.W., and Johnson, M.B. (1989). Woodcock-Johnson psycho-educational battery revised. Texas: DLM Teaching Resources.41. Ylvisaker, M. (Ed) (1985). Head Injury Rehabilitation: Children and Adolescents. San Diego, CA: sen

VI Cognitive Assessment and Intervention

MARK YLVISAKER, PH.D.
BETH URBANCZYK, M.S., CCC–SLP
RONALD C. SAVAGE, ED.D.

Focus:

■ **Cognitive Problems in the Classroom Setting**

■ **Interactions Among Cognitive, Social/Behavioral, and Sensorimotor Needs**

■ **Implications for Team Interaction and Coordination**

■ **Cognitive Assessment**

■ **Interventions for Students with Cognitive Needs**

■ **Language and Communication**

In this manual, the wide diversity of human behavior has been divided into three general categories: cognitive, psychosocial, and sensorimotor. Divisions of this sort are clearly for purposes of exposition only. Lines of demarcation are inevitably blurred and, more importantly, the cognitive, psychosocial, and sensorimotor aspects of human functioning interact dynamically. These interactions, in both normal and impaired functioning, are illustrated in this section. In these discussions of aspects of human behavior, it is essential to hold in sharp relief the total individual who is never adequately described by the distinctions and categories which we use to break large problems into smaller, more manageable problems.

Understood broadly, cognition refers to the intellectual activity involved in the acquisition and use of knowledge, which includes processes such as attending, perceiving, organizing information, remembering, learning, reasoning, and problem solving.

In this chapter, we discuss cognitive disabilities, the ways in which they are manifested in a school setting, how they are assessed and how teachers and other professionals can help the student with a brain injury to compensate for cognitive problems. Attention to cognitive problems is of particular importance following brain injury in children, because cognitive problems are common in this population. Furthermore, cognitive difficulties can result from mild as well as severe injuries in children, and have a profound effect on academic and social growth, but are not always obvious or easy to detect. Failure to detect the cognitive problem may result from the student's performing adequately in school because of the recovery of knowledge and skill acquired before the injury or because the student with frontal lobe injury (the most common kind of injury in closed head injury) performs deceptively well on structure tests of cognitive or academic functioning.

Cognitive Problems in the Classroom Setting

Educators need to approach cognitive assessment and intervention with a useful framework of descriptive categories. An organized, conceptual framework helps to ensure a complete description of students' cognitive strengths and needs, guides exploration of interrelationships among cognitive deficits, helps professionals understand each other's language, and serves as a source of intervention goals and principles of treatment.

Understood broadly, cognition refers to the intellectual activity involved in the acquisition and use of knowledge, which includes processes such as attending, perceiving, organizing information, remembering, learning, reasoning, and problem solving. It is useful to list aspects of cognitive functioning that are important in assessing, describing, and treating cognitive deficits following brain injury and in teaching academic content to students with cognitive disability. These include:

1. The process by which sensory information is taken in, organized, comprehended, stored, retrieved, and used, including attentional processes, perceptual processes, memory/learning processes, and problem-solving processes; and

2. The mental structures that support cognitive processing, including working memory (attentional "space" in which a limited amount of information can be considered at one time), the knowledge base, and the "executive system" (the self-regulatory aspect of cognitive functioning).

Each of these aspects of cognition is explored more thoroughly in Table 6.1, which also includes practical illustrations of problems in cognitive functioning. The categories of cognition and illustrations of cognitive deficits in Table 6.1 include examples that fall most naturally into the province of educators and special educators. In addition, there are examples that will be most familiar to speech-language pathologists, occupational therapists, and psychologists. The need for interdisciplinary programming is supported by the fact that cognitive problems have varied manifestations. Problems with organization, for example, may result in impaired conversational abilities (speech-language pathology), inefficient performance of activities of daily living (occupational therapy), reduced learning efficiency and unfocused classroom behavior (regular and special education), and feelings of frustration or confusion (psychology and social work). There is a cognitive dimension to all activity and all cognitive deficits have wide-ranging consequences. Therefore, all members of the educational team are appropriately considered cognitive specialists and this chapter is intended for the entire team.

Table 6.1:

Possible Cognitive Problems Following Brain Injury in School-Age Children

Aspect of Cognition	Possible Problems Following Brain Injury	Illustration of Problems in a School Setting
Component Cognitive Processes		
attentional processes	■ reduced arousal; sleepiness; fatigue; ■ difficulty focusing attention and filtering out distractions; ■ difficulty maintaining attention; ■ difficulty shifting easily from topic to topic or class to class; ■ difficulty dividing attention between two or more topics or activities.	1. A student may fail to follow the teacher's instruction or comprehend a lesson, not because of a willful failure to attend or an inability to understand, but rather because of an inability to filter out environmental distractions or internal feelings or thoughts. 2. Attentional problems may result in the student talking out of turn, introducing irrelevant topics or responding inappropriately.
perceptual processes	■ difficulty seeing objects in part of the visual field; ■ difficulty perceiving the spatial orientation of objects; ■ difficulty separating the object of perception from background stimuli; ■ difficulty recognizing objects if too much is presented at once or too rapidly; ■ difficulty scanning and visually searching in an organized manner;	1. A student may be unable to do otherwise easy math problems if they are presented on a worksheet page filled with other math problems. 2. A student may be overwhelmed by classrooms that are overly stimulating visually or auditorily. 3. Without a line marker of enlarged print, reading comprehension may appear to be weak.

Aspect of Cognition	Possible Problems Following Brain Injury	Illustration of Problems in a School Setting
memory/learning processes	■ difficulty recalling events from earlier in the day or previous days; ■ difficulty staying oriented to a schedule or to activities; ■ difficulty registering new information or words that have been learned, particularly when under stress; ■ difficulty searching memory in an organized way and retrieving stored information and words.	1. A student may fail to complete assignments, not because of negligence or lack of desire to comply, but rather because the assignment, if not written or repeated several times, is not remembered. 2. A student may miss classes or do assignments incorrectly because of difficulty remaining oriented. 3. A student may require an unexpectedly large number of repetitions to learn simple motor sequences (e.g., tying shoes), classroom routines and rules, and textbook information. 4. A student may need to be reminded to repeat information over and over in order to place it in memory, and to "search memory" in order to find information that has been previously learned, or a student may need compensatory strategies to enhance memory.
organizing processes	■ difficulty analyzing a task into component parts; ■ difficulty seeing relationships (e.g., similarities/differences) among things; ■ difficulty organizing objects into appropriate groups or events into appropriate sequences; ■ difficulty organizing information into larger units (e.g., main ideas or themes); ■ difficulty grasping the major concept from detailed information.	1. A young student, faced with the task of getting ready for gym class, may be unable to break the task into parts and decide what to do first. 2. A high school student may understand each part of a text, but be unable to integrate the information to determine the main ideas and write a short summary. 3. A student may move unexpectedly from topic to topic in conversation because of an unusual set of associations; this may be interpreted as social strangeness or as resulting from a lack of knowledge about the subject.

Aspect of Cognition	Possible Problems Following Brain Injury	Illustration of Problems in a School Setting
reasoning/abstract thinking processes	■ difficulty understanding abstract levels of meaning (e.g., figures of speech, metaphors); ■ difficulty drawing conclusions from facts presented; ■ difficulty considering hypothetical explanations for events.	1. A student who does well with basic mathematical operations may have great difficulty with his/her application in solving word problems or with the more abstract relationships involved in algebra. 2. A student may lose the train of conversation when a figure of speech is used (e.g., "She was climbing the walls.")
problem solving processes	■ difficulty perceiving the exact nature of the problem; ■ difficulty considering information relevant to solving the problems; ■ difficulty considering a variety of possible solutions; ■ difficulty weighing the relative merits of alternative solutions.	1. Having forgotten his/her locker combination and not having ready access to his/her homeroom teacher, a student may simply become upset rather than considering carefully who else may be able to help. 2. Students who fail to comprehend a text with one or two readings may not use strategies to enhance comprehension (e.g., outlining the text, underlining key points, asking themselves questions as they read, discussing the text.)
Component Cognitive Systems		
working memory	■ difficulty holding several words or thoughts or intentions in mind at one time;	1. A student may not be able to follow a 2- or 3- step command, even though comprehension of language is adequate. 2. A student may not be able to think about a compensatory strategy (e.g., "I must repeat this information in order to remember it,") and listen to the presented information at the same time

Aspect of Cognition	Possible Problems Following Brain Injury	Illustration of Problems in a School Setting
knowledge base	■ recall of pre-traumatically acquired information, academic skill, social rules, etc., may have major gaps; islands of preserved high-level knowledge may convey an overly optimistic picture of the student's level; conversely, knowledge gaps at a low level may suggest an overly pessimistic picture of the student's level.	1. Occasionally, a student gains access to pre-traumatically acquired knowledge long after the injury. This may lead the teacher to infer that new learning is occurring at a more rapid rate than is actually the case. Alternatively, the inconsistency in learning rates may lead the teacher to infer that the student is often not trying.
executive system	■ difficulty setting goals; ■ difficulty perceiving strengths and needs in an objective manner; ■ difficulty planning activities; ■ difficulty initiating and/or inhibiting behavior; ■ difficulty monitoring one's own behavior; ■ difficulty evaluating one's own behavior.	1. Students who lack even a rudimentary awareness of current cognitive limitations commonly complain about tasks that are at too low a level and about restrictions on their activity that they perceive as unnecessary. 2. Organized studying (knowing how to divide the task, how to check one's understanding, how to organize the information for easy learning) relies on intact executive functioning, rarely found following severe head injury. 3. Students with initiation problems appear unmotivated and are easily categorized by teachers as resistive, "behavior problems", or as simply lazy. 4. Students who have difficulty monitoring their own behavior and who do not profit from the feedback of others often behave in a socially awkward way.

Educators will note that only a small part of this description of the cognitive mechanism deals directly with the accumulation of academic content (i.e., the knowledge base). Although the learning of academic content is an obvious and important educational goal, educators who work with students with brain injuries must also focus remedial attention on the many cognitive processes which make possible the acquisition of content, and on the executive system, which oversees cognitive activity and allows students to ultimately become independent in their own learning. These intervention themes are expanded later in this section. It is important to note that the teacher's choice is not process versus content. That is, teachers are not expected to postpone teaching academic content while they help students process information more effectively or compensate for ongoing cognitive disability. Rather, teaching academic content is often the ideal context within which to focus on cognitive processes and to help students become more strategic in overall thinking, organizing, remembering, and learning new information.

There are many important interrelationships among the cognitive processes and systems listed in Table 6.1. Impaired organizing processes can, for example, have a negative impact on learning (the better organized information is, the easier it is to learn), on retrieval (an organized search of memory is more efficient than a disorganized search), and on attention (it is easier to attend to details that one organizes into a larger whole). Similarly, a given situation in the classroom may have its basis in a variety of cognitive challenges. The student who fails to follow the teacher's instruction may, for example, have difficulty attending to or comprehending the instruction, or difficulty initiating the appropriate behavior, or difficulty calculating the consequences of not following the instruction.

The results of this approach are inefficiency (at best) and possibly an increase in the fragmentation and confusion that may already dominate the lives of students with too many goals and objectives.

Interactions Among Cognitive, Social/Behavioral, and Sensorimotor Needs

Because difficulties in one sphere of functioning often have implications in other spheres, assessment of children following brain injury must be thorough and systematic. These interactions are illustrated by the following situations:

1. A student who has difficulty remembering task instructions and whose judgment is impaired looks at another student's paper for guidance on how to proceed. This behavior (which is intended as a compensation for cognitive problems) is interpreted by the teacher as cheating. The student is made to stay after school. The punishment is perceived by the student as unfair and a negative behavioral reaction results.

2. A student walks into a lunch room where a group of his friends are laughing at a joke. The child assumes that they are laughing at him, begins to cry, and pushes one of his friends. The situation escalates and the child is suspended from school. Again, in this case, a significant social/behavioral challenge is based on cognitive problems (misinterpretation of the friend's laughter).

3. A student whose physical appearance and abilities were significantly changed by the injury experiences periodic depression, manifested by fatigue, flat affect, and sadness. This compounds the effects of generally weak cognitive functioning on school and social performance, making it more difficult for the child to experience academic or social success. In this case, physical disabilities negatively affect social/behavioral functioning, which in turn further reduces cognitive functioning.

4. A student with impaired right hand function must concentrate so hard on writing that he is not able to listen to the teacher while he is writing. In this way, what is primarily a motor impairment significantly impacts his cognitive functioning. Furthermore, the motor deficit interferes with note taking and thus with the child's ability to compensate for cognitive problems.

5. A student with significantly impaired cognitive functioning may be unable to play gross motor games, like "Hokey Poky," simply because of an inability to follow rapidly presented instructions. Thus, a cognitive problem may look like a motor problem, when in reality no motor problem exists.

6. Many students with mild motor problems can learn to compensate by giving themselves specific instructions (e.g., "Put the heel down before the toe"). However, reduced "space" in working memory may make it impossible to instruct oneself and also do all the other things necessary to navigate a busy hallway. Thus, cognitive problems can interfere in important ways with a child's ability to compensate for motor problems.

However, the cognitive problems that students often experience following brain injury usually persist, despite good recovery in other areas and despite attempts to remediate the difficulties through targeted practice.

Implications for Team Interaction and Coordination

The complexity of cognitive functioning and its interaction with physical and social/behavioral functions mandate careful coordination of the student's total educational and therapeutic program. In a fragmented program, each classroom teacher decides independently which aspects of the child's needs should be stressed, and related service professionals (e.g., speech-language pathologists, occupational therapists, counselors, adaptive physical education teachers) address their own special areas of professional interest without integrating their intervention with other members of the team. The results of this approach are inefficiency (at best) and possibly an increase in the fragmentation and confusion that may already dominate the lives of students with too many goals and objectives. Furthermore, intervention may be at cross-purposes, with one professional promoting compensation for a problem with remedial exercises. Finally, staff who work in isolation fail to exploit daily opportunities to promote generalization of other staff members' objectives.

The student's age, the size and nature of the school, and the number of professionals involved in the program all influence decisions about how to best integrate the cognitive components of the child's program. In elementary school settings, it may be possible to expect the classroom teacher to meet regularly with other professionals and thus manage the student's program as a team. In high school settings, it may be more effective to appoint one person "coordinator" of the total program. This person would be expected to meet regularly with all members of the team to facilitate communication and to promote ongoing problem solving in an attempt to keep the educational program up to date and integrated. Several states (e.g., New York, Iowa) have designated TBI Coordinators and district teams to develop systems of support for students and their families.

The program coordinator must have a good understanding of the consequences of TBI; have a thorough understanding of education law and funding possibilities; be willing to be the student's advocate; be an effective communicator; be supported by the school's administration; be accessible to the team that works with the student and to the family; and have large stores of energy. Furthermore, the coordinator, who may come from inside or outside the school, must work well within an intervention framework that highlights interactions among cognitive, social/behavioral, and physical functioning.

Cognitive Assessment

In this section, we discuss the principles of cognitive assessment that are applicable to educational diagnostic evaluation, to ongoing classroom assessment, and to the assessments conducted by psychologists, speech-language pathologists, occupational therapists, and others interested in the student's cognitive functioning. Because the cognitive profiles of students with brain injuries differ in important ways from profiles of children with congenital learning disabilities or developmental delays, assessment results must be flexibly interpreted. The need for careful interpretation is further supported by the fact that few of the psychological, educational, language, or perceptual tests in common use has been specifically validated for use with students with brain injury.

The selection of assessment techniques depends on the purposes of assessment (see chapter on educational evaluation). Psychologists, educators, and therapists are accustomed to using the results of standardized tests to place students in special programs, to justify services, and in some cases to select objectives of intervention. Great caution must be exercised when tests are used for these purposes with children with brain injury. Depending on the nature of the child's needs, formal tests can either exaggerate or significantly underestimate the extent of the problems.

> **Depending on the nature of the child's needs, formal tests can either exaggerate or significantly underestimate the extent of the problems.**

Students with perceptual and/or motor problems, with severely limited tolerance for frustration, or with strong anxiety reactions may perform worse on tests than their classroom learning behavior would predict, especially if appropriate accommodations have been made in the classroom. Such students may be inappropriately placed in special education classes, despite their potential to succeed in regular classroom settings with certain adaptations and special supports. On the other hand, formal assessment has a number of features that may result in many students with brain injury performing better on testing than would be predicted by the student's very inefficient classroom learning. These features include:

1. The controlled and distraction-free testing environment may compensate for poorly regulated attentional functioning.

2. The use of short tasks and relatively brief testing sessions may compensate for reduced endurance, persistence, and attention span.

3. The use of very clear test instructions and examples may compensate for weak task orientation and impaired flexibility in shifting from one task to another.

4. The use of highly structured tasks and clear instructions to start and stop, may compensate for weak initiation, inhibition, and problem solving.

5. Test items that do not include real-life amounts of information (input or output) or rate of delivery may compensate for weak integration and organization of information and generally reduced efficiency of information processing.

6. The use of tests that do not require the storage and retrieval of new information (not known pre-traumatically) from day to day (or longer periods) may compensate for significant new learning impairment.

7. The encouraging interactive style of the examiner may compensate for the child's inability to cope with interpersonal stress or perception of demands.

8. The basal and ceiling procedures of standardized tests may conceal gaps below basals and surprising strengths above ceilings, common features of brain injury profiles.

Furthermore, many tests (including commonly used intelligence tests) measure skills and information acquired before the injury. Therefore, results from these tests may give a very misleading picture of the student's potential for learning new information and skills. These considerations strongly support the need for informal assessment and diagnostic teaching to complement formal assessment, especially if the goal is to plan intervention and educational programming. This is further supported by the frequent finding that children with brain injury perform inconsistently. Factors that may affect test performance include task demands, setting, familiarity, interest level of the task, and the people in the testing room.

Whether assessment is based on standardized tests or informal diagnostic probes, evaluators must attempt to describe the strategies that the child uses spontaneously to perform tasks, the effects on performance on strategies suggested by the evaluator, the task variables (e.g., how concrete? how simple? how interesting for the child? how cued? what type of materials?), environmental variables (e.g., how quiet? how familiar?), and interactive variables (e.g., how supportive? how motivating?) that are most important in promoting efficient learning and independent problem solving. It is this information, not scores, that guides teaching and other cognitive intervention. In short, there is nothing that can replace a period of active teaching while systematically varying task, environmental, and interactive variables. This type of assessment has come to be discussed under the heading, "dynamic assessment" and is particularly important for students with brain injury because of their confusing profiles.

In interpreting assessment results, consideration must be given to the student's pre-injury learning profile, learning style, and knowledge base. Often students with brain injury have a history of some degree of learning problems. This fact will certainly influence placement and intervention decisions. It is also very important to know if a student pre-injury had a particular strength in an area of functioning that is now impaired. Such students may have to modify previously developed habits that are no longer effective (e.g., expecting to comprehend material on one reading).

Often, graded curricular materials are adequate for the kind of diagnostic detective work that is needed to acquire comprehensive and useful information about the student's cognitive functioning. If tests are used, they may need to be modified in order to examine cognitive and academic processing, particularly if perceptual or motor problems are present. In some states, test modifications are prescribed by law. Modifications may include allowing different response modes, making directions more precise, giving examples, enlarging print, allowing the use of a calculator, reducing the amount of visual information on a page, allowing line markers, and obtaining timed and untimed scores. Reports must describe all modifications used during the testing.

The interpretation of assessment results is further complicated by the need to describe the student's strengths and needs in relation to that student's goals and living and learning environment. Spatial orientation problems, for example, would be debilitating for a student who had to find his own way to school and around a spatially complex environment and whose goal is to become an airline pilot. These problems may be negligible for the child who is bused to school where he spends most of his day in a homeroom. Similarly, functioning at a very concrete level of language and interpretation would be a major problem for a college-bound student, whereas there may be little impact on a student in a vocational track.

Furthermore, the well-known difficulty that many students with brain injury have generalizing skills from one setting to another and from one task to another suggests that a fragmented program will not yield functionally useful results.

Annual achievement tests give useful information about the student's overall knowledge and skill mastery from year to year. Students with brain injury, however, require frequent evaluations of progress in relation to short-term objectives, understanding that progress might be quite inconsistent. Follow-up testing can be used to determine if the student has retained newly learned information over a substantial period of time.

Interventions for Students with Cognitive Needs

In this section, we suggest an approach to intervention that can be used by classroom teachers and other professionals (e.g., speech-language pathologists and occupational therapists). The approach highlights:

1. The development of the student's cognitive skills as well as the teaching of academic content;

2. Methods which teachers can use to compensate for the student's cognitive problems; and

3. Techniques which students can be taught to compensate for their own cognitive problems.

Many books have been written on these subjects and at best we can hope to give illustrations that may stimulate teachers' thinking about how to best structure the educational process for individual students. Although the texts on instruction for students with developmental disabilities may include many methods relevant for children with brain injury, teachers must also remember the differences among these diagnostic groups. Even when IQ scores are within normal limits, the cognitive problems of students with brain injury may be more severe than those of students with learning disabilities and may exist in combinations that are quite unique. For example, children with brain injury may regain many previously acquired academic skills (e.g., reading, writing, and calculation skills). This may make much of the curriculum of the classroom for learning disabilities irrelevant for the students, despite the possibility of perceptual deficits, attention/concentration difficulties, memory problems, comprehension problems, organizational weakness, and self-regulation problems being even more severe than many of their peers with learning disabilities.

Process and Content

The significant cognitive problems resulting from brain injury affect learning in all academic content areas. Although it is customary for school programs and IEPs to focus on teaching academic content and measuring academic progress, it is critical that programs for these students emphasize cognitive processes and social/behavioral functioning in addition to academic content. The goals and objectives for these students should highlight instruction in "learning how to learn" by targeting cognitive problem areas identified during formal and informal evaluation and focusing on their compensation. Similarly, progress for these students should be measured in both traditional academic terms and in terms of their development of cognitive problems in areas such as attention, memory, organization, and problem solving.

Assisting students to process information more efficiently or to compensate for cognitive problems is ideally done using the student's academic content and materials as the context for learning. For example, the social studies textbook can be used as the context for organizational exercises; math worksheets may be the best context for practicing controlled attention or perception. If cognitive processes are targeted in an unfamiliar setting and with unfamiliar materials, improvements may not transfer to functional settings and materials.

More importantly from an intervention perspective, clinicians must engage in creative and structured diagnostic therapy to test hypotheses about which problems are primary and which are secondary and about the most effective intervention strategies.

Compensatory Strategies

In recent years, there has been substantial interest in intervention designed to remediate cognitive problems or at least to improve underlying cognitive skills. Many "cognitive retraining" workbooks and computer programs have been developed that target attentional, perceptual, organizational, and rote memory abilities. There is some evidence that specific cognitive exercises of this sort can result in modest improvements in performance on the tasks used in training.

However, the cognitive problems that students often experience following brain injury usually persist, despite good recovery in other areas and despite attempts to remediate the difficulties through targeted practice. In such cases, teachers and clinicians need to focus their attention on ways to compensate for those problem areas. Compensatory strategies include both 1) procedures that teachers use to structure the environment and learning process for the student to promote adaptive behavior and to maximize learning potential and 2) procedures that students may use to compensate for their own cognitive deficits. Table 6.2 lists several illustrations of how teachers can compensate for specific cognitive needs within a classroom environment and of how they can teach particular students to actively compensate for their own difficulties. Compensatory strategies used by students may include external aids (e.g., tape recorder, log/memory book, a "buddy" system for note taking), overt behavior (e.g., asking the teacher to repeat information or to write it down), and internal procedures (e.g., rehearsing and organizing information to make it easier to remember).

Table 6.2:

Interventions for Students with Cognitive Needs

Selected Aspects of Cognition	Possible Instructional and Compensatory Strategies
attentional processes	■ Gain student's initial attention by connecting new learning to prior knowledge; ■ Use clearly defined objectives that are meaningful for the student; ■ Use short and concise instructions and assignments; ■ Reward on-task behavior; avoid punishing behavior that results from extreme distractibility; ■ Use novel, unusual, relevant or stimulating activities; ■ Provide well-placed rest periods, breaks, or physical activity to minimize the effects of mental fatigue or stamina problems; ■ Closely monitor time of day, medications and fatigue factors; confer with physicians to determine the feasibility of adjusting medication times so as not to conflict with instructional times; ■ Be alert for attentional drifts and redirect the student to task when necessary;

Selected Aspects of Cognition	Possible Instructional and Compensatory Strategies
attentional processes (con.)	■ Explore a variety of cuing systems; (e.g., verbal cues, gestural cues or signs at the study site that remind the student to stay on task); ■ Remove unnecessary distractors in the classroom; ■ Use verbal mediation strategies, such as inserting questions within a lesson, directing attention to the task and topic; ■ In therapy sessions, use tasks specifically designed to help the student focus his/her attention; (e.g., simple maze learning tasks or letter/number cancellation tasks, emphasizing speed, accuracy, and the self-instructions that might promote heightened attention to task); help the student to transfer this improved, self-directed attending skill into the classroom environment.
visual-perceptual processes	■ Describe the visual instructional material in concrete terms; limit the amount of visual information on a page; ■ Provide longer viewing times or repeat viewings when using visual instructional materials; ■ Facilitate a systematic approach to reading by covering parts of the page; ■ Place arrows or cue words, left to right, on the page to oreint the student to space; teach the student to use the cues systematically to scan left to right; ■ Provide large print books or use books on tape; ■ Move the student closer to visual materials or have the materials enlarged; ■ Place materials within the student's best visual field; consult with an opthalmogist; optometrist or occupational therapist about possible visual-perceptual problems.

Selected Aspects of Cognition	Possible Instructional and Compensatory Strategies
auditory-perceptual processes	■ Limit the amount of information presented; give the student instructions or other verbal information in appropriately small units; ■ Present verbal information at a relatively slow pace, with appropriate pauses for processing time and with repetition if necessary; ■ State information in concrete terms; use pictures or visual symbols if necessary. ■ Have the student sit close to the teacher, with an unobstructed view; ■ Teach the student to ask questions about the instructions or materials presented, to ensure comprehension; ■ Teach the student to request slower or repeated presentations if the material is presented too rapidly.
memory/learning processes	■ Try to make the material to be learned significant and relevant to the student; ■ Match the student's learning style (e.g., visual learner) with the instructional method; ■ Give meaning to rote data to enhance comprehension and learning; ■ Regularly summarize information as it is being taught; ■ Give multisensory presentations; ■ Reinforce information presented with pictures or other visual images; ■ Control the amount of information presented at one time; ■ Use overlapping techniques, such as repetition and rehearsal; ■ Have the student overlearn material; ■ Couple new information with previously learned information; ■ Teach the student note-taking techniques; ■ Teach the student to use a datebook for appointments, assignments, and other important information; ■ Teach the student to use one or more of the following techniques: visual imagery, "chunking" techniques (organizing information into easily retrieved segments), association techniques, mnemonic devices, such as acronyms, repetition and rehearsal techniques or adaptive devices such as appointment books, calendars, alarm watches and tape recorders.

Selected Aspects of Cognition	Possible Instructional and Compensatory Strategies
organizing processes	■ Provide an organizing template that the student can use to add information to; ■ Limit the number of steps in a task; ■ Provide part of a sequence and have the student finish it; ■ Give cues, such as "Good, now what would you do?"; ■ Structure thinking processes graphically, (e.g., with time lines, outlines, flow charts, graphs); ■ Use categories to focus on one topic at a time; ■ Identify the main idea and supporting details; categorize the details (e.g., using who, what, when, where and why questions); teach the student to do the same when reading or listening to lecture material; ■ Teach the student to practice organizational skills at home (e.g., an organizational system for school material and daily routine).
problem-solving processes	■ Develop a problem-solving guide to help students through the stages of problem solving (e.g., identify the problem; acquire relevant information for solving the problem; generate several possible solutions; list pros and cons for each solution; identify the best solution; create a plan of action; evaluate the effectiveness of the plan); ■ Raise questions about alternatives and consequences; ■ Allow the student to bring up relevant real-life problems that are appropriate for group discussion; promote brain-storming about alternative solutions and their usefulness; ■ Introduce roadblocks and complications to enhance "detouring" skills and to encourage flexibility; ■ Provide ongoing, non-judgmental feedback. ■ Break large tasks into sequences of smaller tasks; provide the student with a checklist to keep himself on task.

Because of the many factors that affect the success of strategy intervention, teachers must thoroughly consider a student's eligibility for this approach. Children in the early grades may not be the best candidates, because these students lack adequate awareness of their own cognitive processes (metacognitive awareness) and consequently cannot be expected to easily learn techniques to compensate for difficulties in these processes. Or, more likely, they might learn the technique as rote behavior, but not understand the purpose of the technique or situations in which it is applicable, and therefore not generalize the skill. The same considerations apply to older children who are very impaired cognitively.

However, prerequisites for mature strategic behavior should be targeted in young children and those with significant impairment. This includes intensive efforts to help children (1) understand which tasks are hard and which are easy, (2) understand that there are special things that can be done if a task is hard and (3) improve problem-solving behavior in the context of concrete everyday problems.

Similarly, children who have extremely restricted attentional abilities, who are very impulsive, or who do not have goals to which the compensatory strategies are relevant may not profit from strategy intervention. Students who are shy or very self-conscious about their disability may be able to learn strategic behaviors, but may not use them for fear of making themselves stand out. Finally, if there is not consistency in encouraging the student's use of specific strategies from classroom to classroom and therapy session to therapy session within that student's school program, then strategy intervention will likely fail, despite otherwise good potential for the student to profit from this approach.

In the presence of any of these issues that affect the success of strategy intervention, teachers should address the issue as part of a holistic package of intervention designed to improve strategic thinking and strategic behavior. In many cases, teachers can determine whether a student is a good candidate for strategy intervention only by attempting to teach a strategy. Initially, a significant amount of time is required to teach the strategy and its importance. Cueing systems must be developed to remind the student to use the technique. The goal is to have the student use the strategy when appropriate and without external cues. Generalization to functional settings and activities is, therefore, an essential component of the instructional process. This includes using the student's classroom materials as the instructional medium and teaching the strategy in the context of classroom activities. Students who cannot be taught to compensate for their own cognitive problems can still be assisted in their learning by the teacher's creative use of compensatory methods of instruction and environmental structuring. Some students whose performance improves when they use compensatory procedures (e.g., outlining material when reading) may need reminders indefinitely to use the procedure, because the student may lack initiation or adequate awareness of the nature of the disability.

It is important for teachers to invite and assist older children and adolescents to become participants in the problem solving and decision making that go into educational planning. If students can be helped to understand the obstacles to their academic success, to see current school problems in relation to important goals that they espouse, and to generate solutions and strategies for themselves, the intervention will very likely be much more effective and the student will, at the same time, develop autonomy and independence.

Table 6.3 presents a breakdown of problem-solving skills in terms of a sequence of stages of deliberate problem solving. Teachers can use this as a guide to working through educational programming with selected students, with the goal of developing a negotiated educational plan that the student sees as personally meaningful and as a product of his/her own problem solving. This guide, or a simplified version of it, could also be taught to selected students to use when they face difficulties, in or out of school, which require thoughtful solutions. The more students are given control over their own instructional process, the greater the likelihood that they will be actively engaged in and will benefit from that process.

Whether treatment gains are achieved by means of retraining or compensation, it is essential to promote generalization of skills by systematically varying the context and task. In most cases, it is programmatically more effective for the language specialist to work in the classroom jointly with the educator, or, if this is impossible, in a consulting capacity. This enables the student to practice skills and strategies in the context of their desired use and with materials that are academically relevant. Generalization and maintenance are threatened if speech and language pathologists, or other ancillary staff, restrict their therapeutic activities to settings, materials, and tasks that are unique to that specific therapy. Teaching or therapy that is not functional or is done in isolation only exacerbates preexisting problems for the student.

Communication and Language

In this chapter, we have emphasized the importance of integrating the educational and therapeutic services for children following severe brain injury. The rationale for this integration of services includes the observation that cognitive problems experienced by many of these students have similar implications for the work of teachers, psychologists, speech and language pathologists, occupational therapists, counselors, recreation therapists, and others. Furthermore, the well-known difficulty that many students with brain injury have generalizing skills from one setting to another and from one task to another suggests that a fragmented program will not yield functionally useful results. All professionals on the team need to engage in assessment and intervention activities in a way that is not tightly integrated within a total program that has functional, interdisciplinary goals.

Since cognitive-communication problems are very common after a brain injury, the following section outlines some particular areas that professionals need to recognize. There is vast literature available to speech and language pathologists, for example, that deals with intervention for students with cognitive-communicative disability and illustrates the application of our cognitive framework to one of the supports in a school setting and recommends ways in which support services (not just language and communication therapy) can be integrated into the student's total educational program. The intervention literature in the field of developmental language problems has become increasingly relevant to the cognitive-communicative problems associated with brain injury. In particular, intervention discussion that focus on discourse and thought organization, word retrieval, and social skills should be of interest to clinicians working with students with brain injury.

Language Problems:

Except in the early, acute stages of recovery, deficits specific to linguistic processing are not common following brain injury in children. Unlike many adults with aphasia following stroke and children with specific congenital language problems, students frequently recover the surface features of the linguistic code (e.g., syntax, morphology, and phonology) and have little difficulty understanding or producing words and sentences in an age-appropriate manner in nonstressful situations. Those children who do have specific language problems are generally identified—either because their problems are obvious in conversation or because language tests in most common use are designed to identify these problems—and can be treated by speech and language pathologists with intervention techniques appropriate to specific language problems.

The more common language and communication problems following brain injury are, unfortunately, also harder to detect—typically based on cognitive and/or social/behavioral challenges—and can have serious negative effects on the student's academic performance and social functioning. While comprehension of spoken and written language may appear to be intact under ideal conditions and with manageable amounts of language to process, this can be and typically is very misleading. With increases in the rate at which language is presented, in the amount of language presented , in the complexity or abstractness of the language, in the environmental distracters, and in the level of stress attached to a task, comprehension and retention of information frequently deteriorate much more rapidly than would be expected. For example, a seventh grade student may score at a seventh grade level on tests of single work or sentence reading comprehension, but have severe comprehension and retention problems when asked to read an entire chapter in a seventh grade text or to read in a busy classroom environment.

Expressively, students with brain injury frequently struggle for the right words to express their thoughts and ideas and speak in ways that may be well-organized at the sentence level, but are very disorganized and tangential at the level of longer discourse (spoken or written). These problems are often the reflection in language of general inefficiency in information processing, of generally disorganized thinking, or of pervasive attentional problems. They can have significant effects on academic performance and achievement.

Conversational interaction is vulnerable following brain injury as a result of the combined effect of cognitive weakness and social/behavioral problems. Students may produce language that is unacceptable to the setting and situation (because of impulsiveness or impaired social judgment), wander unpredictably in conversation, fail to initiate interactions or have difficulty inhibiting unacceptable statements. These common difficulties in the pragmatic domain of language typically cause the child with brain injury to seem "different"—socially awkward—and to lose friends.

Language Assessment:

Students with brain injury present a complex diagnostic dilemma for the speech and language pathologist. There are no standardized tests or assessment batteries designed to probe all of the areas of likely language dysfunction following brain injury. Clinicians must, therefore, combine tests with careful observation of language and communication behavior in a variety of settings and contexts and with carefully designed probes that reveal the possible effects of cognitive and social/behavioral problems. More importantly from an intervention perspective, clinicians must engage in creative and structured diagnostic therapy to test hypotheses about which problems are primary and which are secondary and about the most effective intervention strategies.

Social interaction skills, including conversational competencies, can be assessed using one of the available protocols for observing the pragmatic aspects of language. Observations should include variation in key factors, including large and small groups, and familiar and unfamiliar settings, partners and topics. The effects of cognitive stress can be explored with customized probes that systematically vary one of the cognitive stress factors at a time. For example, the effects on language comprehension of processing inefficiency can be assessed by presenting two narratives that are matched in every way but the variable under investigation (e.g., length, rate of presentation, or environmental distractions). Analogous probes can be used to explore expressive functioning. Results of these probes should be compared with assessments in other disciplines since the weaknesses being explored rarely affect language alone.

Summary

This chapter has described a variety of cognitive and communicative needs that are common following brain injury in children. Impaired cognitive functioning, even if subtle, can have far-reaching effects in a demanding academic setting. Because of the often unusual patterns of strengths, needs and preferences in the students, the emphasis has been upon classroom observation and diagnostic teaching as the keys to assessment. Intervention must be customized for each student. In most cases, however, appropriate classroom adaptations and compensatory strategies are part of the intervention package.

Also stressed are the interconnections among cognitive, social/behavioral, and sensorimotor functioning. Indeed, it is often the social and emotional consequences of cognitive deficits that are most problematic for parents and teachers.

Contributed by Susan Pearson

David

According to his parents, David exhibited normal developmental milestones prior to his injury at age 16 months, when he was run over by a tractor on the family's farm. Initially, there was no loss of consciousness. He was taken to a local emergency room where he was stabilized and then transferred to a nearby trauma center. A head CAT scan revealed a right basilar skull fracture and pneumocephaly. An abdominal CAT scan revealed a small liver laceration. Three days after the injury, David's mental status deteriorated and he had a tonic-clonic seizure. Magnetic Resonance Imaging (MRI) revealed what appeared to be hemorrhages; intracranial pressure remained normal. Seizures were controlled with phenobarbitol. Approximately ten days after the initial injury, David was transferred to a facility for rehabilitation. On the day of admission, David was spiking temperatures and it was believed that he had developed pneumococcal septicemia and meningitis. He was treated with a 14-day course of antibiotics. At the time of discharge from rehabilitation, his diagnosis included: basilar skull fracture with left cerebral infract; right hemiparesis; traumatic optic neuropathy, right eye; seizure disorder. David was discharged on January 11th and on January 15th, his parents met with rehabilitation staff and the pre-school department from the local education agency to review his current status and needs and to plan appropriate home intervention follow-up services. During this meeting, it was determined that David should receive weekly services including instruction from a home intervention teacher and therapy in the areas of speech and physical therapy.

An outpatient follow-up evaluation was conducted approximately three months after discharge. Updated information from the family and local education personnel indicated that the family was adjusting nicely to having David home from the hospital and that they had good support from members of their extended family. David's mother indicated that the older brothers were resentful at times of the attention given to David. David's parents were encouraged to have the boys talk about their feelings, which were normal reactions to the situation. The parents were also encouraged to have their older son get involved with a local sibling support group. David's cognitive abilities were assessed to be at approximately a 13-month level (CA 20 months); expressive language abilities at an 8-month level. Follow up evaluations were conducted approximately two months later, with some minor improvement in these scores. Approximately one year post injury, David continued to receive homebound services from the local education agency. Plans were being made to involve him in a center-based preschool developmental classroom (physical disability) three days per week in the fall.

Evaluations at one year post injury showed continued progress in speech (approximately three months gain in six months time). Cognitive testing showed that David responded most consistently to items at the 14-15-month level (CA 29 months). Phenobarbitol continued to be used for management of seizures.

David was evaluated six months later, (summer) prior to the school year. Receptive and expressive language abilities were assessed informally to be at a 22-24-month level. David had been learning to "sign" to communicate some of his needs but it was noted that his ability to do so was severely compromised by his overall neuromotor involvement. It was suggested that a total communication approach including manual communication, communication boards and oral speech might be the most successful approach. The Introtalker was suggested as an appropriate communication device for David to use as it allowed the teacher to pre-record desired responses according to specific lessons. It was also recommended that David maintain his current speech/language therapist for the sake of consistency and rapport and that speech/language services be given high priority in his schedule. Cognitive testing indicated skills to be at the 24-26-month level (CA 36 months).

At the end of the first semester of center based preschool it was decided that David needed more individualized attention and the decision was made to move him to a new preschool with fewer children. David's mother reported that David would receive speech/language services twice a week in the new setting. The local physical therapist would continue to provide range of motion activities at school. The Introtalker was being loaned to the preschool developmental classroom from approximately one month fro David to use on a trial basis.

During the fall semester of the following school year, an outpatient evaluation indicated a need for dietary management of weight gain. At CA 50 months, fine motor skills were at the 19-month age level with minimal use of the right hand and a local evaluation/consultation was recommended. Receptive language was at 32 months; expressive at 24 months. The staff suggested that an augmentative communication evaluation would be appropriate. David had been demonstrating some use of the Introtalker and was also using vocalizations, gestures, pointing and signing to communicate. AFOs were recommended to keep his foot in a more neutral position for walking and weight bearing. David's cognitive skills were slightly below the three year level at this time. David's teachers voiced frustration with the Introtalker and viewed it as "inflexible". David's teachers felt the Zygo Macaw might be more appropriate and planned a trial with that device. Recommendations from the evaluation included: continue intense speech/language services to develop a multimodal expressive system; encourage and reinforce speech attempts; continue to use picture symbol communication boards, experimenting with the size and placement of pictures to accommodate any visual difficulties; continue exploring options for a voice output communication aid; provide practice on the adapted classroom computer which could provide the opportunity for the development of talking word boards in the future.

School personnel report excellent communication with David's parents and feel his parents are good advocates for David. David's problems with attention and his inability to express himself are his teachers' greatest concerns. The teachers also feel that David's developmental level contributes to his resistance of help and his desire to do things independently.

VII Social/Behavioral Aspects of Brain Injury

ANN V. DEATON, PH. D.
RONALD C. SAVAGE, ED.D.
L. JEANNE FRYER, PH.D.
ELLEN LEHR, PH.D

Focus:

■ **Social/Behavioral Issues in the Classroom**

■ **Assessment**

■ **Intervention**

■ **Guidelines for Managing Challenging Behaviors**

Social Behavioral Issues in the Classroom

Social/behavioral skills are frequently impaired as a consequence of brain injury. When a student re-enters school these behaviors are often stumbling blocks that interfere with appropriate behavior in the classroom and during extracurricular activities, interaction with the teacher and other students, as well as in taking advantage of the educational curriculum offered. Programming for social/behavioral skills must be as carefully attended to as cognitive and sensorimotor skills following brain injury. This requires an interactive working environment with teacher, counselor, student, family, and other team members all participating to ensure adaptive re-entry and on-going performance in the school setting.

The behavior patterns that emerge after injury are unique to each individual child or adolescent.

Socialization occurs as an interactive process influenced by genetic disposition, environmental conditions, cognitive development, and social/effective maturation. When this process flows smoothly, effective, age-appropriate social behavior can be engaged in by the individual. However, after a brain injury this interactive process is disrupted. The factors that may be involved in the alteration of social/behavioral skills after brain injury include:

■ age at time of brain injury;

■ location of the area of brain dysfunction;

■ severity of the brain damage and length of coma;

■ time elapse since the injury occurred;

■ pre-existing intellectual aptitudes;

■ pre-existing personality characteristics;

■ type of environment pre- and post-injury;

■ motivation for recovery/improvement;

■ nature of family, including changes in interaction and relationships post-injury.

The behavior patterns that emerge after injury are unique to each individual child or adolescent. However, likely consequences of brain injury consist of reduced self-control of behavior, less effective use of social skills, and impaired social development. The actual expression of social/behavioral aspects of brain injury varies widely. Preschool and primary school aged children are more likely to show overt hyperactivity, distractibility, impulsivity, and temper tantrums after injury. However, this is not always the case and many children's primary difficulties after injury may be seen in reduced initiative and sparsity of behavior, rather than in behavioral excesses. Older children and adolescents are more likely to have difficulty inhibiting their behavior, often expressed through irritability, agitation, and inappropriate comment, and are more likely to complain of somatic effects such as headaches and fatigue. In extreme circumstances, behavioral effects in adolescents can also include antisocial behaviors, drug and alcohol abuse, and sexual misconduct.

Children and adolescents who have been functioning adequately pre-injury are sometimes less likely to develop social/behavioral difficulties post-injury than those children and adolescents who already were experiencing difficulties in these areas before their brain injuries. However, even children and adolescents who were functioning well in social/behavioral areas pre-injury are at increased risk for developing new difficulties in these areas. It is also important to remember that social/behavioral difficulties related to brain injuries often do not appear until many months and sometimes even a year or more post-injury.

Cognitive aspects of brain injury play a large part in impaired social interaction. In order for a student to be socially competent he/she must be able to assess a situation, be sensitive to other people and their needs as well as his/her own, discriminate among social cues, review a course of social action, anticipate possible consequences of his/her actions, decide what is appropriate, and act on decisions. Ylvisaker, et al. (1994) list a number of cognitive factors that are involved in impaired social competence following brain injury:

■ poor awareness and perception of social and communicative events

■ inadequate retrieval of rules of social interaction

■ reduced ability to take alternative perspectives

■ disorganization at the level of introducing, maintaining,
and terminating topics of conversation

■ disinhibition and weak self-monitoring of verbal and nonverbal behavior
which may result in the student:

■ repeating information,

■ making inappropriate and offensive remarks,

■ demonstrating reduced comprehension,

■ appearing uninterested or unmotivated.

When social skills (those interpersonal behaviors that contribute to an individual's effectiveness as part of a group) are impaired or not developed, the socialization process is altered and maladaptive social interaction is likely to occur. Consequently, social behavior after brain injury often becomes a function of:

■ organic factors (impulsiveness, inappropriate comments and actions, confusion,
emotional lability, misperceptions of intent, lack of awareness of deficit);

■ personality factors (obsessiveness, social deceptiveness, rigidity, tolerance, hardworking);

■ environmental factors (family conditions, community/school expectations)

Age appropriate use of social skills also depends on secure emotional development. Disrupted emotional development can lead to social/behavioral problems in the school and community setting. Emotional development is based on the ability to:

■ devote energy to self, (e.g., understand one's own needs; differentiate inner needs from environmental demands);

■ care about self, (e.g., be aware of personal care and emotional needs);

■ explore environment, (e.g., attend to detail; be aware of others; be responsive to others);

■ be honest with self, (e.g., understand the consequences of personal actions on others;
evaluate one's own performance);

■ take risks, (e.g., try new tasks appropriately).

Each of these elements develops along a continuum and interacts with each of the other elements as the child moves towards maturity. The possible alteration in these elements and their effect on social/behavioral functioning must be considered when working with students after brain injury. The outcome of alterations in social/behavioral functioning post-injury is often seen in increased social isolation, loss of pre-injury friends, and difficulty in making new friends.

It is important to realize that following brain injury, subtle and sometimes dramatic sequelae alter not only the student's acquired skills and learning ability, but also the individual's perception of self as well. Children and adolescents can be keenly aware that they have altered abilities after brain injury. They may experience marked frustration and depression when attempting to be like they were prior to injury, and react with anger and grief for their losses. Adolescents, especially, experience these changes as a loss of self-confidence that interferes with their age-appropriate identity development. Children and adolescents often describe these feelings as "being out of control" or feeling "crazy." Students need to have a clear explanation of how their feelings are related to their brain injury, their "right" to be angry or sad about the changes in themselves, and the confidence that other people understand their problems and will help them surmount their difficulties.

Children and adolescents often describe these feelings as "being out of control" or feeling "crazy."

There are several areas of social/behavioral functioning to consider in planning educational programs for students after brain injury. Within the school environment, students must be able to attend, remember information, carry out plans of action, and integrate new skills and tasks into appropriate behaviors. These are social, as well as cognitive tasks. Students also need to be able to control their emotions, have a reasonable frustration tolerance level, initiate appropriate behavior, express empathy for others, and regulate and control their own behavior.

Assessment

It is important to assess the organic, personality, and environmental factors with respect to a student's overall social/behavioral functioning in order to best understand the impact of the brain injury on an individual. Comparison of the student's behavior and capacity pre- and post-injury is important in highlighting the changes that have occurred, both those directly related to injury effects and in reaction to the effects. Probably the most accurate method of determining these changes is by interviewing the student's parents, siblings, and friends. The student him/herself may, at least initially, be less aware of social/behavioral changes than of more obvious physical or sensorimotor changes. The comparison of others' reports, the student's reports, and findings from the evaluation can indicate the student's needs in social/behavioral areas. Assessment of the student must include evaluation approaches that identify cognitive, personal, and group competencies related to social/behavioral functioning.

Necessary cognitive competencies which are a part of social/behavioral functioning include:
■ **Attention/discrimination:** Ability to monitor the environment and to differentiate salient from unimportant information.

■ **Memory:** Ability to remember previously learned information with or without external cues.

■ **Communication:** A person's ability to send and receive information about basic and complex needs and ideas.

■ **Ability to Learn:** Ability to make use of information in a replicable fashion and ability to alter that behavior as a result of the information and the environment.

■ **Judgment:** Ability to perceive and understand the environment in such a way as to maintain one's own and others' safety.

Necessary personal competencies include:
■ **Self-regulation/behavioral control:** Ability to monitor and control one's own behavior in relationship to a code of behavior and in relationship to the immediate environment.

■ **Emotional control:** Ability to experience and express appropriate affect in a socially acceptable manner.

■ **Self Respect:** Feeling comfortable about self in relationship to one's values and the values of others; seeing oneself as a unique person separate from others.

■ **Endurance:** Ability to persist in an individual physical activity or in an entire day's physical activity plan, without deterioration of performance competencies due to fatigue.

■ **Grooming and Hygiene:** Awareness of, concern for, and attention to bodily appearance, bodily health.

■ **Sexuality:** Awareness of male and female sexual traits, seeing oneself as attractive and acceptable to others.

■ **Structuring Time:** Ability to structure time appropriately to meet both work and social/recreational/leisure needs.

Necessary group competencies include:

■ **Identification with the group:** Ability to perceive how unique personal needs and skills are allied with other group members to help maintain the group.

■ **Asking for help:** Ability to feel comfortable enough with oneself to be able to communicate one's need for assistance in such a manner as to encourage those asked to provide the requested help.

■ **Friendship/support skills:** Ability to know what friendship means and to demonstrate through words and actions emotional investment in other individuals and the group.

Intervention

Generally, in order to facilitate positive socialization and continued social/behavioral development of students after brain injury within a school setting, one may choose to:

■ Change the individual (teach new skills, re-learn old skills);

■ Change the environment (provide more structure, limit stressors, control social interactions, provide adult supervision);

■ Provide functional adaptations (provide reminders regarding behavioral expectations, teach methods to increase self monitoring of behavior, teach friends to give appropriate feedback about behavior).

Intervention with students who have experienced brain injury frequently requires adaptation and creative problem solving, along with a great deal of structure. Patience and a calm, controlled demeanor are imperative, as models of behavior for the student, as well as to facilitate one's own ability to deal with the variable behaviors that may occur as a consequence of brain injury. Consistency of approach builds a sense of control for the student and also enhances his/her learning of social and behavioral skills. Acknowledging and then redirecting the student's behavior away from the problem at hand (frustration with task, inappropriate verbalizations, angry outbursts) is a useful technique, especially in the period shortly after injury or with those students who had severe injuries. Such students are often very suggestible. However, they are also likely to be quite perseverative, so one may have to redirect frequently.

In teaching or re-teaching appropriate social skills and increased behavioral control with students post-injury, an instructional model may be helpful. Given the behavior characteristics of brain injury (distractability, poor memory, impulsiveness, disinhibition, poor generalization, lack of initiation, etc.), the model of reconstructive education on the next page suggested by Luria (1974) has been very successful in working with these students. This model consists of six steps:

Model for Reconstructive Education

1. Stating the goal - sharing the end point
Example: the goal—restoring appropriate social interaction with peers; the end point—being able to interact with one student appropriately in a structured activity.

2. Identify task specific to disability
Example: the task—playing a broad game with one other student demonstrating ability to abide by the rules, take turns, and win or lose gracefully.

3. Reduce task to a hierarchy of activities - Specify each part of task
Example: the hierarchy of activities—choose a game that can be played by two people, read the rules, set out the playing pieces and other game materials, rehearse the game procedures alone or with an adult, role-play social situations that are likely to cause difficulty for the student, model appropriate behaviors in reaction to these situations.

4. Remove external cues and modeling
Example: play the game with another student, initially with adult supervision and coaching, then only with the two students present.

5. Chart progress
Example: have the student record the length of time he/she has been able to play the game with another student appropriately, keep track of the kinds of difficulty the student has with the task (not being able to maintain focus on the game, difficulty tolerating set-backs or losing).

6. Re-evaluate
Example: evaluate progress with the student by discussing/charting any specific difficulties with playing the game and interacting through this means with another student.

Behavioral analysis is another way of learning to manage behavior. The way behavior is described can determine the way people feel about the student who displays such behavior. A functional analysis of a specific behavior is a way of objectively observing it and will lead to a clearer understanding of how to alter or modify it. A careful, complete understanding of why the behavior is occurring is most useful in determining effective interventions. In order to accomplish this, educators and students can often collaborate in describing and recording behavior according to the following:

- **the conditions which exist just before the behavior occurs (antecedents to the behavior); and**
- **the specific characteristics of the behavior itself:**
    - is it directed at somebody or something, or in response to a specific event?
    - how frequently does it occur?
    - how long does it last?
    - how intense is it, what affects the level of intensity?
    - is there a pattern to the occurrence?

Once the behavior has been identified and described, an approach to manage or change the behavior can begin. Substituting a desired behavior and increasing its occurrence must be done along with decreasing the undesired behavior. The basic principles to remember are:
■ work on identifying the steps to acquiring and utilizing the positive behavior and reward them as they occur;
■ record the increased frequency of positive behaviors and give the student direct feedback about his/her success;
■ when negative behavior occurs:
■ ignore it,
■ distract/substitute another behavior,
■ remove the student from the situation.

It is important to reiterate that much of what is seen as social/behavioral aspects of functioning are influenced by both cognitive and physical abilities. For example, students may exhibit inappropriate behaviors because of memory problems resulting in an inability to remember rules or the consequences of their actions. Specific neurological components of injury may directly influence behavioral control and emotional expression. It is critical that all involved be aware of the social implications of such impairments so they can be viewed and dealt with in the proper perspective.

There are several specific types of behavior that appear consistently as a consequence of brain injury and can be very disruptive to the educational process. Some of these behaviors and suggestions for intervention strategies are highlighted on the next page. A more thorough understanding of these behaviors should allow for careful planning of their management and thus will help reduce socially maladaptive behavior.

Table 7.1

Guidelines for Managing Behaviors

Behaviors Intervention Strategies	Possible Instructional and Compensatory Strategies
secondary depression and withdrawal	■ While students often have memory problems, they do not generally forget what they wanted "to be" before their injury. Hence, depression after a brain injury is common for many students as they adjust. ■ Teachers need to help students recognize the things they can do rather than what they cannot do. Keep students involved with the "real world". ■ Be an "active listener" for students who need to talk and focus on the positive feelings the student displays. Use caution when dealing with family matters or matters that are very sensitive. However, let the student's counselor know of these situations so they can be addressed. ■ If a student becomes suicidal or expresses such, contact the school psychologist and/or counselor and the parents/guardians immediately.

Behaviors Intervention Strategies	Possible Instructional and Compensatory Strategies
lack of insight/denial of disabilities	■ Many students with right hemisphere injuries may not recognize their problems and, hence, deny that they have any. ■ Speak to the student in terms of "strengths and needs" rather than disabilities or deficits. Try to get the student to verbalize his/her needs rather than just "see" his/her inabilities. ■ Find the student's strongest learning modality (visual, auditory, tactile) and use this modality to help the student recognize his/her problem areas.
impulsive behavior/lack of inhibition	■ Students with frontal lobe injuries often feel "out of control" and cannot effectively inhibit impulses. ■ Staff need to help students better manage their worlds by keeping activities organized and structured. Use calendars, schedules, time clocks, etc., to help students orient to the world around them. ■ Key words/phrases help students track their behaviors and lessen impulsivity. Merely asking a student "why" he/she did something does not help the person control those actions. ■ Have students write down their plans as much as possible. Check their daily journals and focus the students on routines to decrease "not knowing what to do next" behaviors.
poor emotional control	■ The key to handling poor emotional control is to redirect behavior, change the subject/environment, and refocus the student's attention on something positive. ■ Student's are often very sensitive to negative criticism and often react strongly if they feel someone is making fun of them. Use humor positively and not as a way to ridicule or embarrass students. ■ Mood swings are common after brain injury since the brain is having difficulty trying to inhibit impulses and respond properly to emotions. Teachers need to reorient students to positive goals and help them recognize that normal recovery, like life, is full of "ups and downs." ■ With some brain injuries, students may lose the ability to feel guilt and empathy. They may use offensive language and become very critical of others. Teachers need to respond to students by saying, "When you talk like that it makes ME very uncomfortable" rather than reprimanding the student. Show the students how they might better state what they are feeling in a more positive tone.

Behaviors Intervention Strategies	Possible Instructional and Compensatory Strategies
apathetic/not caring attitude	■ Give students a choice between doing one thing or another, do not give them a choice between doing something or doing nothing. Keep the students involved with each other, group interaction helps to reduce apathy. ■ Help the student explore what it is he/she really wants, proceed in small steps, set easy goals, and show the student he/she can succeed. ■ Structure practice situations so the student can practice perceiving the feelings of others or how to respond appropriately.
agitation and irrability	■ Agitation and irritability are usually not purposeful, but more often the result of something else - fatigue, frustration, "bad days" - which are often not recognized by the student. Help the student pinpoint what is wrong and then find ways to cope. ■ When a student becomes agitated/irritated and has an outburst, REDIRECT the student away from the source of frustration. Do not dwell on the outburst or what the student did. ■ During severe outbursts, redirect and reduce the stimulation or frustration by offering the student an alternative action. Take the student for a walk, to the gym, or have the student do something physical to "work it off."
aggression	■ Students who become aggressive have generally been agitated for a period of time prior to an aggressive display. It is important to know your students well enough to redirect agitated behaviors by heading them off before the student explodes. Keep the student's counselor informed of behaviors that you feel could become harmful. ■ Speak very calmly and gently to a student who has become aggressive. Even if the student is screaming, raising your voice will only make matters worse. You need to act as a "role model" for the student - be a calm, caring and controlled role model. ■ Use key phrases which are familiar to the student to help him/her gain control of the aggressive behaviors. If the student needs to work out physically, take him/her to a gym or some other safe place. ■ If the student's aggressive behavior cannot be controlled and/or threatens the safety of staff or other clients, the teacher needs to follow the school's emergency procedures. However, use a teaching model, not a punishment model.

Children and adolescents may also need intervention focused on helping them to adjust to the changes they have undergone because of their brain injuries. Students have experienced a truly severe injury that can affect all areas of their functioning and jeopardize their future development. The emotional stress of this is often prolonged and can be overwhelming. If it is not sensitively handled, psychological crises can be precipitated by what otherwise would be routine events. For example, graduating from high school can be emotionally painful if the effects of a brain injury have caused a student to alter his/her plans to attend college or to train for a specific career. Intervention specifically focused on emotional coping with brain injury effects can be beneficial, either on an individual basis or through a support group with other children or adolescents who have shared this experience.

In summary, the social/behavioral aspects of brain injuries in children and adolescents are critical components that can restrict their ability to engage effectively in learning and social interaction in the school setting. Educators are in a unique position to be able to accurately assess and intervene in order to minimize the effect of social/behavioral difficulties post-injury in their students. As in all areas of the student's management, though, a team approach is essential in fully understanding the neurological, emotional, cognitive, and environmental aspects of specific social/behavioral challenges following brain injury.

See Social Skills Intervention Bibliography in Reference Section, page 182 of this Manual.

VIII Sensorimotor and Physical Factors in Traumatic Brain Injury

MARTIN D. WEAVER, M.D., ED.M.

Focus:
■ **Recovery**
■ **Sensory Motor Deficits**
    Weakness
    Tone
    ■ **Hypertonicity**
    ■ **Hypotonicity**
    Neuromuscular Control
    ■ **Sensory Function**
    ■ **Perceptual Motor**
    ■ **Motor Planning and Initiation**
    ■ **Coordination**
■ **Summary**

Recovery

It should be understood that therapeutic intervention does not actually reverse neurologic pathology in the student with brain injury. Therapeutic intervention quite simply optimizes the functional outcome of natural recovery and maturation. When dealing with a student who has sustained a traumatic brain injury, one must also keep in mind the many variables of recovery that relate to the inciting event. Such variables include age at the time of incident, premorbid functional abilities, site and extent of pathology, as well-related sequelae.

In general there is presently thought to be a much greater potential for recovery following traumatic brain injury than previously believed. Many cases have reported prolonged recovery as well as delayed recovery. Thus, it should be kept in mind that the potential for continued recovery may exist years after the initial insult.

It is hypothesized that uninjured parts of the central nervous system take over the function of damaged areas.

Several theories exist as to the etiology of brain injury recovery. A few of these theories include brain plasticity, neuronal sprouting, and diaschisis. Plasticity refers to the pleuropotential ability of the central nervous system. It is hypothesized that uninjured parts of the central nervous system take over the function of damaged areas. It should be kept in mind that age is an important factor in this theory. Brain plasticity appears to decrease with increasing age. It is thought that there is a progressively irreversible commitment of parts of the central nervous system to specific functions as a person ages. Neuronal sprouting in simplistic terms is the growth of normal neuronal axons to replace axons which were damage due to the injury. There is also said to be re-growth of damaged axons. The growth of these neuronal axons are in an attempt to connect synaptic networks damaged by the traumatic brain injury. Diaschisis is simply the return of function of parts of the central nervous system which are said to have undergone a period of shock secondary to the traumatic injury. These are areas without direct pathology which underwent temporary shutdown due to diffuse effects of the inciting event.

Sensory Motor Deficits

Physiological and anatomical lesions sustained by the student with traumatic brain injury result in several neurological disorders within both the sensory and motor systems. These culminate in disturbances of motoric behavior. Such disturbances include voluntary movement, abnormalities of tone, and neuromuscular control. An understanding of these disturbances and their relation to physical functioning should aid the educator in dealing with a student with a traumatic brain injury.

Weakness

Weakness is a disorder of voluntary movement. The ability to generate muscle tension is known as strength. Power is the generation of muscle tension or strength over time. It is this latter term power which is functionally relevant in describing weakness. Weakness in general can be considered the inability to contract a specific muscle in an extremity with normal power. It presents as the inability to generate muscle tension. A distinction should be made between focal and diffuse weakness. Focal weakness from a central injury as with the student with TBI will have a different prognosis than that resulting from peripheral nerve injury.

Lack of motor strength is described as either paresis or paralysis. Paralysis is the total or complete absence of motor strength while paresis is the partial absence of motor strength. Paresis is usually accompanied by abnormalities in tone. In dealing with paresis it is more useful from a functional stand point to interpret muscle weakness in terms of functional muscle groupings such as hip flexors knee extensors, etc., thus relating the pathology to its impairment and corresponding functional disability.

Weakness often being accompanied by muscular atrophy and decreased range of motion can result in contractures. It is therefore quite obvious how weakness or its complications can lead to difficulty in activities of daily living and overall mobility. The combination of therapeutic exercise including range of motion and positioning techniques through developmental sequencing will foster the student's overall ability. Subsequently, neuromuscular facilitation and strengthening will improve muscular function and enable the student to be more independent in ADL's and ambulation.

Tone

Motor disability may also be due to abnormal muscle tone. It is important to differentiate between hypertonicity and hypotonicity. These two major types of muscle tone abnormalities vary greatly in their treatment and functional implications.

Hypertonicity

Under hypertonicity there are two types of motor dysfunction; rigidity and spasticity. Rigidity is noted when there is an increase in tone through out the range of motion of that extremity. The student with rigidity exhibits co-contractions of the agonistic and antagonistic musculature. Such co-contraction can be exhibited with movement or at rest. When dealing with a student with hypertonicity several factors should be kept in mind, including the level of task difficulty, the child's mental state of alertness and orientation, and any modifications of sensory input including proprioception, vestibular, and tactile senses. Any and all of these factors can affect the student's muscle tone and therefore voluntary motoric behavior. Thus classroom manipulation of sensory input can help decrease hypertonicity and increase function. Individualized modifications to control various factors should be part of the student's educational program. Spasticity is noted when a student displays an increased resistance of muscle to passive stretch. There may be increased muscle stretch reflexes as well as clonus. Spasticity is noted to vary with posture. Although a student may not appear to be spastic in a supine position, extreme spasticity may be noted in an upright standing position.

It should be kept in mind that a certain degree of increased muscle tone, be it rigidity or spasticity, might be helpful for a given student with TBI who has functional disability. Transfers, standing and ambulation training might significantly benefit from a functional degree of increased tone. On the other hand, hypertonicity usually limits joint range of motion with subsequent contracture formation and joint deformity. Asymmetrically increased tone about the axial-skeleton might progress to abnormalities of the spine such as scoliosis. Difficulties with ADL's and mobility might be noted with progressive abnormal posturing, making the student's body handling difficult for caretakers.

Discomfort related to increased muscle tone might interfere with a student's cognition. When dealing with the spastic student it is important to note that nociceptive stimuli tend to increase spasticity. Such irritating stimuli frequently encountered include poor fitting cast, heterotopic ossification, ingrown toe nails, decubiti, bowel impaction, urinary retention, and infection. Pharmacological treatment of spasticity should be in conjunction with more conservative therapeutic interventions. A commonly used antispasmodic is baclofen, as well as diazepam and dantrolene sodium. Following pharmacological intervention accepted treatment includes peripheral nerve blocks utilizing local

When dealing with a student with hypertonicity several factors should be kept in mind, including the level of task difficulty, the child's mental state of alertness and orientation, and any modifications of sensory input including proprioception, vestibular, and tactile senses.

anesthetics. Temporary anesthetic blocks are utilized initially to evaluate functional improvement. Should targeted tone reduction be of benefit, then a more long-term peripheral nerve block is completed utilizing percutaneous phenol.

Hypotonicity

Hypotonicity is best understood as a decreased resistance of muscle tissue to passive stretch. The student with TBI who has hypotonia usually reflects cerebellar pathology. Although not as problematic as hypertonia, hypotonia causes a variety of functional dilemmas. A flaccid extremity might be accompanied by circulatory problems resulting in dependent edema. Shoulder joint subluxation with associated pain is also a complication of hypotonia. Trunk instability may cause difficulty in posture, positioning, and mobility. Ambulatory dysfunction might also result from specific abnormalities such as Genu Recurvatum and foot drop due to decreased tone. Therapeutic intervention should facilitate muscle activity while protecting extremities and preventing joint deformity.

Neuromuscular Control

Neuromuscular control involves the complex integration of sensory and perceptual motor skills combined with the executive functions of motoric planning and initiation. Harmonious synchrony of these functions results in well coordinated purposeful movements.

Sensory Function

Normal functioning requires consistent sensory motor integration. Proper movement necessitates mainly three intact sensory systems which include vision, vestibular, and proprioceptive systems. Students may be able to compensate when one of these sensory systems is damaged, but they are unable to do so when two of these systems are not adequately functioning. Smooth voluntary motoric response necessitates consistent reciprocation between movement and intact sensory systems. The area of the brain known as the post-central gyrus is responsible for interpreting sensory input. Input into this area of the sensory cortex is via the thalamus and internal capsule. Damage to any of these structures could render the student unable to properly interpret cutaneous sensation such as light touch, pressure, temperature, pain, vibration, and tactile discrimination. Due to such abnormal sensory input there may be inadequate sensory motor integration with a resultant lack of coordinated smooth voluntary motoric responses during mobility and activities of daily living.

Perceptual Motor

Additional deficit in sensory motor integration can be brought on by inadequate perception in a student with a brain injury. Such perceptual motor impairments can occur without alternation of strength, tone, or sensation. A major such perceptual motor impairment is apraxia, which is most frequently seen with damage to the dominant hemisphere in the region of the parietal lobe. Apraxia renders a student unable to exhibit known or familiar gestures through or in response to verbal command. There is difficulty in the programming and execution of learned volitional motoric behavior. There are various functional implications of apraxia including apraxia of gate and oromotor apraxia. There are also various types of apraxia including ideomotor, constructional, and ideational. Apraxia can render a student motorically inept, interfering with utilization of every day objects such a tooth brush or cup. Apraxia may be so severe that the student is maximally dependent for activities of daily living.

Motor Planning and Initiation

Prior to a voluntary motoric act there must be the planning of a complex motor sequence following the conception of an action which is preceded by the decision to act. The final step being initiation of the voluntary motor behavior. Students with traumatic brain injury may have difficulty with such initiation and planning. Disorders of initiation include preservation, akinesia, and catalepsy. Perseveration is the inappropriate repetition of a specific motor act. Akinesia or hypokinesia is the lack of spontaneous movement due to difficulty in initiation. Catalepsy is long term maintenance of abnormal postures without change in muscle tone. Catalepsy and akinesia are thought to be due to pathology of the basal ganglia, whereas perseveration results from pre-frontal cerebral pathology.

Coordination

Coordination or control of skilled purposeful movements is often affected in the TBI student. It should also be kept in mind that impaired coordination might often be confused with weakness or tone abnormalities. Disorders of coordination without weakness or tone abnormalities are usually the result of cerebellar dysfunction. Abnormalities in gate or posture usually point to pathology of the cerebellar vermis. Coordination might also be impaired by damage to the sub-cortical motor areas also known as the extra-pyramidal system which includes the basal-ganglia. Involvement of the basal-ganglia will cause impaired coordination known as chorea. The student with TBI may exhibit abnormal involuntary posturing or movements. This is usually due to the lack of cortical inhibition or control over sub-cortical structures. It must be kept in mind that abnormal involuntary movements do not always denote cerebral pathology but may simply reflect pharmacological side effects in students with TBI. Most true abnormal involuntary movements are exacerbated by stress and tend to subside.

> It must be kept in mind that abnormal involuntary movements do not always denote cerebral pathology but may simply reflect pharmacological side effects in students with TBI.

Summary

Students with severe traumatic brain injury usually spend several months in acute hospitalization. This is usually followed by an average of three months of in-patient rehabilitation. An additional half to one-and-one-half years might be spent in various subacute or community based centers. Subsequently most TBI patients become long term students in educational and vocational programs.

Students with traumatic brain injury may suffer from a myriad of sensory and motor deficits. These deficits are due to central nervous system pathology and lead to impairments within, but not limited to, the neurological and musculoskeletal systems. Such impairments render the student with significant functional disability. Such disability leads to students with mild to severe and profoundly handicaps. It is thus extremely beneficial for educators to attempt to understand the aforementioned complex effects of isolated sensory and motor deficits on everyday functioning.

IX Transitioning the Student with Brain Injury from School to Employment, Post-Secondary Education and Independent Living

THERESA KRANKOWSKI, ED.S., C.R.C, C.V.E.

Students with brain injuries experience many dimensions of transition throughout the course of their lives. These transitions may include the movement from hospital to school; teacher to teacher; one therapist to another; regular education to special education; or junior high school to senior high school. Thus, transition must not be viewed as "a single event in time" but an ongoing process which occurs throughout the course of a person's life. Therefore, parents must play an active role early on in assisting their son or daughter to prepare for his/her future. The importance of advocacy, planning, preparation, and knowledge of resources are all critical aspects of preparing students with brain injury for adult life.

In order to effectively advocate for your child's future plans after high school, awareness of the present legislative initiatives under the 1990 Individual with Disabilities Education Act (IDEA) is vitally important. This law mandates that "every eligible student have transition services incorporated into his or her individual education plan (IEP) no later than age sixteen, and when appropriate, beginning at age 14 or younger." Also important is a statement of interagency responsibilities or linkages that is clearly delineated in the IEP before the student leaves the school setting.

IDEA defines transition as follows:

A coordinated set of activities for a student with an outcome-oriented process which promotes movement from school to post-school activities including:

■ Post-secondary Education
■ Vocational Training
■ Employment (Competitive and Supported)
■ Continuing and Adult Education
■ Independent Living
■ Community Participation

As a result of a student's possible long-term need for services, it is essential that the transition process begin as early as possible. Many times school systems wait until the student is 21 or 22 to begin this process and as a result, the complexities of the student's post-vocational or educational plans remain unaddressed. Advocating for services at an earlier stage can ensure that the student's needs have been well thought out and long-term supports secured. Planning and preparation are essential to designing an effective transition plan. Therefore, this next section will highlight important components needed in the plan.

The involvement of a vocational rehabilitation counselor is key. This professional, employed by the Department of Vocational Rehabilitation Services, is responsible for assisting the student in identifying long-term career goals, exploring academic and vocational plans both during and after high school. However, to develop a more focused and specific vocational plan, a school-based vocational assessment is essential. This type of assessment, a second key in the process, can guide the student and counselor when developing and implementing the vocational plan. A school-based vocational assessment provides information regarding the student's academic and vocational skill strengths, needs, and accommodations/strategies. We must closely review these assessment results in order to ensure both accuracy in the findings and to determine if it truly reflects the student's strengths and needs. Overall, a quality vocational assessment should indicate whether the student's career choices are commensurate with his or her abilities.

In order to effectively advocate for your child's future plans after high school, awareness of the present legislative initiatives under the 1990 Individual with Disabilities Education Act (IDEA) is vitally important.

In conjunction with a vocational assessment, supervised work experiences are another significant part of the student's transition plan. Here, the vocational counselor can gain a better understanding of the student's challenges with executive functioning and how such challenges may significantly impact his or her ability to formulate career goals, carry out vocational related plans, and monitor one's work performance. Therefore, supervised work experiences provide students with several learning opportunities: 1) to practice critical job seeking and keeping skills; 2) to determine compensatory strategies which can be utilized on an independent basis; 3) to gain insight into strengths and areas of need; and 4) to self monitor work performance and accurately assess abilities. Finally, through these work experiences, the skills of students may be validated and thus warrant the need for post-secondary education.

Depending upon the student's capabilities or career goals, post-secondary education could be an integral part of the student's transition plan. If the student demonstrates academic potential, consider a two-year, junior or community college as well as a four-year institution. This type of transition requires a specific detailed outline highlighting information regarding acceptance criteria, necessary supports available on campus, and how the student pursues his or her major course of study. Other critical issues to consider before the student enters a post-secondary include: specific services available for students with brain injuries; knowledgeable professionals who can educate university personnel about the student's impairments and the impact on academic performance; and finally, arrangements that need to be made to establish both living and academic accommodations.

The student's transition plan must provide information on what needs to occur to assist with achieving his or her maximum level of independence.

Preparation for the student to move from a dependent living situation to independence will require both knowledge and access to resources. The student's transition plan must provide information on what needs to occur to assist with achieving his or her maximum level of independence. In this respect, parents need to work collaboratively with educators by reinforcing at home what the student learns in school. For example, at school, the student may be learning budgeting and banking skills. At home parents can reinforce this by having their son or daughter establish his or her own bank account, manage finances, and take responsibility for paying bills. The student's capability to carry out these life skills in natural settings will be valuable information for school personnel in linking the student with the appropriate independent living options and support. These supports may include one or more of the following: case management services; attendant services; medical services; and transportation. Important to note is that without one or more of these supports the student's residential stability could be jeopardized — resulting in a negative impact on other life areas such as work, school, and social activities.

A final part of the student's plan involves establishing linkages with adult service providers. The quality of life and extent to which students with brain injuries achieve the desired goals of employment, post-secondary education, and community living are dependent upon the effectiveness of cooperative planning and availability of adult services. Adult service representatives such as vocational rehabilitation counselors, social security representatives, and residential service providers play an integral role in facilitating the student's successful transition. Representatives from these agencies must take into account the student's needs and preferences, and must actively seek their input in the decision-making process. Adult service providers need to work collaboratively with the interdisciplinary team and provide information on: the type and kind of services available through the agency; requirements to qualify for services; availability for services at the local level; and procedures for completing applications. Overall, the goal of this cooperative effort is to strive for a holistic approach to service delivery, looking at the entire person rather than dividing the individual into frigid functions or disciplines.

In summary, transition planning is a vital part of assisting students with brain injuries to identify their present and future academic potential as well as strategies to address the complexity of their needs. Effective transition plans require timely, coordinated efforts of educators, rehabilitation personnel, parents and students as their own advocates in determining their future employment, post-secondary training, and independent living. In essence, the transition process provides students with brain injuries an opportunity to restore their "loss of self" through gains of self knowledge, self advocacy, and self determination.

References

Brown, D., Hiltenbrand, D., and Jones, E. (1989). Project PACT: Partnerships in Action for Community Transition. Career Education for Special Needs Individuals: Learning, Earning, and Contributing. Division on Career Development, (pp. 241-252).

Condeluci, A., Cooperson, S., and Seif, B. (1987). Independent Living Settings and Supports. In M. Ylvisaker and E. M. Gobble (Ed.S.), Community Reentry for Head Injured Adults, Boston, MA: College Hill Press.

Krankowski, T., (1993). Meeting the Transition and Post-secondary Needs of Students with TBI. Special Topic Report, #1, 1-8.

West, L., Corbey, S., Stephens, B.A., Jones, B., Miller, R. J., Wircenski, M. S. (1992). Integrating Transition Plans Into the IEP Process, Reston, VA: Council for Exceptional Children.

Contributed by Susan Pearson

Evan

Evan was 15 years old when he developed what appeared to be a viral illness characterized by fever, fatigue and diarrhea. Approximately two weeks later he was admitted to the Intensive Care Unit for evaluation of a persistent febrile illness complicated by aphasia, right hemiparesis, and altered mental status. He had a temperature of 106∫. Evan apparently had a bacterial infection in his heart which resulted in blood clots that caused a left hemispheric stroke. Prior to his illness, Evan was a healthy young man who was developing normally. He had been involved in all regular education classes and had completed the eighth grade. School reports indicated that he was an average student who had some minor difficulty in the area of math.

Evan remained in the hospital for approximately six weeks and was then discharged home, where he lives with his parents and twelve year old brother. His mother stated that "what happened to Evan, happened to all of us," and shared that she was feeling guilty about Evan's illness. Evan's younger brother was also having a difficult time adjusting to the changes in his older brother. Evan's mother was not sure whether this was "normal" adolescence or if it was a reaction to Evan's illness. By report, Evan's behavior has changed since the stroke. His mother feels he is not as outgoing socially as he was before and voiced concerns about his emotions and behavior.

At a follow-up evaluation after hospital discharge, Evan was found to be about 25 pounds underweight, and was described as wan, emaciated and fatigued. Evaluation by a speech/language pathologist indicated that his volume, rhythm, rate and intonation had been affected and that his production of words was sometimes indistinct. Social language skills and grammatical sentence structure were intact and age appropriate but pronunciation of multi-syllabic words was problematic and he was sometimes difficult to understand.

Cognitive testing revealed intellectual abilities in the average – high average range although he was noted to have some difficulty with tests specific to short-term memory. Visual motor tasks also appeared to be problematic. On a test requiring mental flexibility and categorization skills, Evan experienced significant difficulty. Academic testing indicated that Evan's skills were in the average-high average range with the exception of math and spelling. Although Evan frequently recognized when something was spelled incorrectly, he was not able to problem-solve to correct it, which tended to be very frustrating for him. Writing was extremely tiring and time consuming. During the evaluation, Evan presented himself as a sincere, concerned and somewhat anxious young man. Staff felt that he was not yet physically ready to return to school and recommended homebound instruction until his stamina improved; consultation with a speech/language pathologist from the local education agency; counseling for Evan to assist him in working through his feelings; a sibling support group for his younger brother; and a high calorie diet to gain weight. Staff consulted with the homebound instructor to assist in setting up Evan's program at home.

Approximately two months later during a second follow-up evaluation it was suggested that Evan return to school on a part-time basis. His strength and endurance had increased significantly, he was no longer napping in the afternoon and had gained five pounds. There was still some mild weakness on his right side, but his gait had improved. Cognitive testing indicated improved mental flexibility and organization but Evan continued to show difficulty with word retrieval. His academic performance was similar to the previous evaluation with significant weaknesses in handwriting and math. Before Evan returned, medical and educational personnel held a staffing to determine Evan's specific needs. Staff recommended that Evan's weight be monitored on a weekly basis by the school nurse and that speech/language services be provided to help improve his word pronunciation, word finding and organization of verbal discourse. It was determined that Evan's workload should be limited to two courses and that adaptations be made for written expression because of physical fatigue and spelling problems. School personnel were encouraged to provide assistance with organization and to consider extended year programming during the summer. A case manager, the school guidance counselor, was identified to facilitate communication between all involved and to be available to Evan as needed during the school day. Family counseling was also suggested.

Over the next two months, Evan had returned to school part-time and his stamina had continued to improve. Plans were made to have him start back to school full-time at the beginning of the second semester. Evan's mother reported that she was less anxious about him and that he had become more independent.

After Evan returned to school full-time, school personnel reported some problems with attendance. Teachers were feeling that they would not be able to credit Evan for course work because of the amount of time he was missing. After checking with the family, it was determined that Evan was experiencing some sleep disturbance and having trouble getting back to sleep. As a result, Evan was coming to school fatigued or staying home to sleep. Evan's mother was encouraged to have Evan attend school and take naps there if necessary. She acknowledged that this had been difficult for her to enforce as she was worried about Evan becoming ill again.

During the second semester, Evan's cardiologist gave him permission to return to physical education, but indicated that he should not be involved in contact sports, and that he should be allowed to rest as needed.

X Promoting Health and Wellness for Students with Brain Injuries

MONA WHITMAN, R.N., M.ED.
RONALD C. SAVAGE, ED.D.

Introduction

Health is more than the absence of illness. It is holistic, ever changing, and a dynamic condition. Wellness is more than health. It requires deliberate action. Promoting health and wellness for children and adolescents with brain injury takes teamwork. The nature, manifestations, recovery patterns, and characteristics of brain injury are oftentimes perplexing and confusing. Understanding our roles in the recognition, recovery, and reintegration of these students demands knowledge and expertise. To see clearly we must stay in focus. We must see each student as an individual with unique skills and abilities. We must weave what "was," "is" and "will be" into a life tapestry of productive and satisfying possibilities.

The Three R's–
Recognition, Recovery, and Reintegration

Familiarity with the medical/health, physical, psychosocial, developmental, cognitive/communicative, and behavioral aspects of brain injury provides an essential foundation for our role as educators, team members, and advocates. For those professionals unfamiliar with medical terminology, pharmacology, and the intimate relationship between physiology and behavior the effects of brain injury can seem quite perplexing. It is not unusual for families, teachers, siblings, and peers to feel overwhelmed and helpless because of the complex interrelationships among common sequela of brain injury: the high variability in recovery patterns, the sensitivity of developmental and age-related maturational effects on delayed manifestations, the astonishing incongruity and variation in performance capabilities, and the multiple popular misconceptions and erroneous assumptions propagated through the media "soap opera" depictions of time-lapsed recovery from coma to community. It is no wonder that people arrive in the midst of a catastrophic incident with conflicting expectations and perspectives. It is no surprise that there remain numerous misconceptions about the nature of brain injury on the part of otherwise well-informed, intentioned, and educated people as a result of the conflicting messages and experiences they may have historically received through narrative recounts of personal experiences or exposure to the interpretation of film and media.

However, the school nurse is in an excellent position to improve public and community awareness through education, prevention, advocacy and clarification of misconceptions people may have about brain injury. Table 1. clarifies some common misunderstandings.

Table 1

Facts About Brain Injury

■ Brain injury occurs after birth and is the leading cause of death and disability for children, adolescents and young adults.

■ Brain injury affects the person injured, their family, friends and peers.

■ The only cure for brain injury is prevention.

■ Children do not just "bounce back" after brain injury.

■ Problems from brain injury may not show up until much later on when the child reaches later developmental stages.

■ Recovery from brain injury is not a one-time event; it is a life-long process.

For those professionals unfamiliar with medical terminology, pharmacology, and the intimate relationship between physiology and behavior the effects of acquired brain injury can seem quite perplexing.

The First "R": Recognition

Recognition begins with understanding the definitions, nature, incidence, manifestations, and outcomes associated with acquired brain injury. Oftentimes, the confusion inherent in medical, educational and rehabilitation definitions can lead to misinterpretation, inappropriate placement, misdirected interventions or lack of recognition (BIA, 1990; Savage, 1991). By providing a clear framework health care professionals can assist others to better understand the nature and consequences of brain injuries "acquired" after birth.

Types of brain injury:

Considerable variation exists in the terminology and definitions used to describe brain injury. The nurse and the child's physician can help others by providing a basic working knowledge of the subject. Firstly, brain injury occurs after birth. It may result from a traumatic event (e.g., fall, assault, car collision, etc.) or a nontraumatic event (e.g., drowning, choking, toxic poisoning, etc.). Damage can occur from diffuse disruption (e.g., shearing, stretching and tearing of the neurons from a sudden impact) or local injury from bleeding or bruising (e.g., hematomas, contusion). The incidence of shearing injuries is higher in children than adults, while brain contusions appear to be less common in children (Zimmerman & Bilaniuk,1978).

Injuries with a skull fracture are referred to as open head injuries (OHI) and those without are called closed head injuries (CHI). Skull fractures are more common in infants. Direct damages from the immediate injury are known as the " primary effects " and those occurring shortly after the injury such as swelling, shifting or further bleeding (e.g., increased intracranial pressure, herniation, or hematoma) are known as "secondary effects."

Incidence of brain injury:

Statistics from The National Pediatric Trauma Registry (1994) and The Brain Injury Association (1994) indicate that injury is the leading cause of death and disability for children and young adults. Brain injury is the most frequently recorded diagnosis in the pediatric registry. Children between 5-9 years of age were reported to have the highest incidence of injury followed by those 1-4 years old. Infants under one year were the third highest age group reported to be injured noting that 64% of infant injuries were due to child abuse. Adolescents ages 15-19 years were particularly vulnerable to motor vehicle collisions.

When the registry's statistics were adjusted to account for age distribution, their findings were consistent with the Brain Injury Association's, citing motor vehicle collisions as the leading cause of injury. However, falls were the most frequent cause of injury for children with 20% of the children having fallen 8 feet or more. Falls from windows were found to be seasonal with 80% of the falls occurring between April and September. Young children often fell from furniture or down stairs in walkers.

The next largest category of causes for injury in children was motor vehicle related collisions where children were either occupants in the car or hit by a car as a pedestrian or while bicycling. A large number of children with injuries were not wearing protective restraints such as child safety seats or seatbelts and if bicycling were not wearing helmets. The facts are alarming. While public awareness has improved in recent years, considerable attention and effort still needs to be placed on public education regarding the scope, magnitude, and consequences of brain injury in children and

> Brain injury is the most frequently recorded diagnosis in the pediatric registry.

adolescents. The school nurse in particular can play a pivotal role in addressing these education and advocacy needs by developing informative presentations and materials on topics pertinent to brain injury for students, parents, teachers, and the community.

Levels of severity:

While the terms mild, moderate, and severe brain injury are frequently used to describe the "type" of injury the child sustained, these same descriptors often fail to tell us about outcome. Since children are less likely to lose consciousness after a blow to the head they are often thought to have fully recovered within days and weeks. However, over time children may experience significant cognitive and/or behavioral problems after only a minor blow to the head. In addition, as one searches the medical literature, there is no consistent definition for mild, moderate, or severe brain injury among physicians, psychologists, educators, etc. (Eichelberger et al., 1990).

Mild brain injury:

Seventy percent (70%) of all brain injuries are classified as mild (BIA, 1994). Mild brain injury may or may not involve loss of consciousness. In the mildest form the person has momentary confusion and disorientation that may resolve completely within a matter of seconds after the event. They may not be able to remember the impact or what happened immediately before the incident (retrograde amnesia). This type of injury usually resolves without further sequelae except for some degree of permanent retrograde amnesia. Some individuals experiencing mild brain injury may also forget what happened immediately after the injury (post-traumatic amnesia) and their confusion may extend to minutes rather than seconds.

Most children with mild brain injuries experience a good recovery, however, 1-3% of these individuals may develop complications such as bleeding or swelling, requiring neurosurgical intervention (Dacey and Dikmen, 1989). Many children may continue to have post-concussive symptoms such as headache, fatigue, concentration/attention problems, dizziness, or blurred vision for up to three months after the initial injury.

Children respond to mild brain injury differently than adults. Initially after the injury, they demonstrate more pronounced physical responses such as lethargy, nausea, and vomiting (Snoeck et al., 1987). Therefore, vigilant observation and assessment is essential to detect subtle changes that may herald deterioration and serious complications.

Additionally, there are some individuals who will continue to experience persistent difficulties following a seemingly minor injury. Parents and teachers need to be aware of signs that may indicate persistent problems requiring attention such as any increases over the pre-injury baseline for fatigue, unexpected absences, inattentiveness, difficulty remembering, conflicts with peers, inappropriate or disrespectful behaviors (Ylvisaker and Savage, 1994).

The role of the health care professionals in the prevention, detection, assessment and management of mild brain injury is considerable. Taking the lead in the design and implementation of safety training programs, inservice education presentations, development of assessment checklists, follow-up observation tools, and tracking forms for early detection of performance problems, etc. can have a considerable impact on improving the quality of services and interventions offered in the school for these students and families. Coordination and integration with local hospital emergency rooms, physician offices, child care centers, etc. can foster continuity in protocols and improved detection, appropriate recognition and treatment, community-wide.

Children respond to mild brain injury differently than adults.

Moderate brain injury:

Those with moderate brain injuries experience a loss of consciousness and post-traumatic amnesia which usually subsides and resolves completely within 24 hours post-injury. Moderate brain injury is less common than mild or severe. While most individuals with moderate brain injury go on to experience a good recovery, many may be left with longstanding pronounced cognitive and psychosocial problems.

These individuals are particularly vulnerable because their quick dramatic hospital recovery (i.e., going from being unconsciousness to waking up and following commands within 24 hours) is such a relief that it oftentimes leads to false sense of security. The individuals seem quite well overall, but problems may develop later on when they are confronted with the demands of returning to home, school and the community.

Severe brain injury:

Severe brain injury results in loss of consciousness which may last for days, weeks, or months. Initially, the child may only move in response to deep pain. He/she may have signs of brainstem damage such as posturing and abnormal pupillary reactions. The child's hospital course may be complicated by the need for additional surgeries because of hematomas or increased intracranial pressure. The incidence of hematomas is lower for children than adults, but more children with severe brain injury have increased intracranial pressure (Shapiro & Marmarou, 1982; Bruce et al., 1978).

Severe brain injury may also result in blood pressure, heart rate, breathing and temperature regulation problems and seizures. Children tend to develop early seizures more frequently than adults, but that does not necessarily mean that the child will develop post- traumatic epilepsy (Shapiro, 1987).

A person with severe brain injury overcomes serious life-threatening obstacles sometimes against all odds. Early in a person's recovery, he/she may struggle to recognize people, places and things. As the individual progresses and his/her confusion lessens, he/she learns or relearns how to eat, drink, move and communicate. Parents, friends and family are thrust unexpectedly into the strange and unfamiliar sights and sounds of intensive care, traveling through the ups and downs of an often times rocky rehabilitation course, and, finally, arriving at the point they have been longing for— returning home. And returning home is another step in the child's ongoing recovery. Recovery is not a single event, it is a life-time process.

The Second "R": Recovery

Recovery for students with brain injuries may be more complicated than it is for adults. A child's brain is still developing and the impact that a brain injury can have on a developing brain is relatively unknown (Savage, 1994). However, many children experience life-long problems growing up with a brain injury (Klonoff et al., 1993) as the world becomes more challenging and their brains have been compromised by an earlier injury.

Predicting outcome:

Outcome has many different meanings. For those in research it may mean isolating factors with strong predictive recovery value. For those in large trauma centers it may mean the prospect for survival and discharge from the hospital. For those in rehabilitation centers it may mean the type of permanent limitations expected to confront individuals as they re-enter the community.

A person with severe brain injury overcomes serious life-threatening obstacles sometimes against all odds.

Many professionals have investigated outcome following brain injury. Yet, despite considerable effort, precise understanding of the frequency of expected disability from severe and moderate brain injury is uncertain and the extent of residual problems experienced by persons with good recovery is not well documented (Savage and Wolcott, 1994; Jennett & Teasdale 1981; Gianotta et al. 1982; Levin et al. 1982; Kraus, 1987).

Prediction of outcome in children is even more difficult since it requires determining the effects of injury on a growing and maturing brain. Moreover, as the complexity of learning increases with subsequent developmental stages, problems may not emerge until much later on when the child is asked to use advanced cognitive, social and physical skills (Ylvisaker and Savage, 1994). Understanding the impact of brain injury requires a knowledge of brain function and maturation, human growth and development, and the common characteristics of recovery.

There is an intense interplay between problems in one area with those in other areas.

Physiology and function:

A basic understanding of brain anatomy, physiology, function, and development is essential for accurate problem identification, goal setting, and selection of appropriate strategies aimed at promoting optimal recovery (Savage, 1994; Bigler, 1993). Generally speaking, the brain can be thought of as having three major components: the brainstem, cerebrum, and cerebellum. The brainstem regulates vital body functions such as arousal, primitive response to pain, temperature, blood pressure, heart rate, and respiration. The cerebrum governs sensation, voluntary movement, perception, visual interpretation, motor and sensory function, language, organization, and problem solving. The cerebellum exerts control over coordination of movement.

Children's brains mature in growth spurts that closely follow their major developmental stages (Savage, 1994; Lehr and Savage, 1989). During ages 1 through 6 all regions of the brain experience synchronous development as the child learns to manipulate and use objects, form words, and put things in serial order. From the ages of 6 to 10, as the child begins to perform simple operation functions such as understanding the meaning of phrases like my "mother's brother" or mastering the concept of weight, there is a pronounced acceleration of development in the sensorimotor areas of the brain. At ages 10 through 13 the visual and auditory areas of the brain take the lead and the child now begins to master formal operation functions such as calculations. In the early teen years from 13 to 17 the brain masterfully sculpts connections between the visuoauditory, visuospatial and somatic areas, accelerating hormonal and emotional development and allowing for the emergence of dialectic abilities such as analysis, critique, and rebuttal. The final stages occur from ages 17 to 21 with full development of the frontal executive systems of the brain and the refinement of abstract reasoning and hypothesis formation.

Potential problems:

Students with brain injuries may experience a wide range of physical/health, cognitive/communicative, psychosocial and behavioral problems (Savage and Wolcott, 1994, 1988; Ylvisaker, 1989; Blosser and Depompei, 1990). Physical problems may include muscle spasms and tightness, weakness, paralysis, tremor, uncoordinated or slow movement and poor balance. Visual problems such as double vision, neglect of one side of the visual field, and blurred vision may be present. Cognitive difficulties may include memory problems, poor attention, concentration, and organization, distractibility, lack of initiation, and impaired problem solving. Slowed or slurred speech, word finding difficulties, or incorrect word usage may impair communication. Poor self-concept, self-esteem, loneliness, isolation and frustration may lead to psychosocial adjustment difficulties. Behavioral inappropriateness, impulsivity, social awkwardness, and poor interpersonal skills may hamper socialization and relationship formation (Feeney and Urbanczyk, 1992).

There is an intense interplay between problems in one area with those in other areas. Cognitive difficulties may affect physical performance. For example, an inability to understand or remember the instructions may result in poor performance on tasks requiring motor sequencing. Physical limitations may affect cognitive performance. Poor coordination may hamper notetaking or painful muscle spasms may result in distraction and diminished concentration and attention. Cognitive problems may be misinterpreted as behavioral problems. Impaired initiative, memory deficits and poor recall may result in the person being labelled as lazy, noncompliant, or stubborn. Behavioral difficulties may result in psychosocial problems such as alienation, frustration, depression, and substance abuse.

Patterns of performance:

Students with brain injuries may continue to change neurologically for weeks, months, and even years after their return to school. These changes may be rapid or may occur slowly over time. Considerable variation exists in the range of disabilities experienced by persons with brain injuries. Individual physical, cognitive and behavioral disabilities may be mild, but, overall, may combine to produce severe disability. Academic profiles may be varied and "gappy" showing excellent performance and preservation of high level knowledge skill coupled with gaps in lower level areas (Ylvisaker, 1990). Performance on standardized and formal testing is usually better than actual day to day performance. Prior successful learning strategies may have to be "unlearned" because they are no longer effective. There may be marked discrepancies between the person's perception of his/her ability and his/her actual performance capability. This may be compounded by a lack of recognition of performance deficits. Significant variations in performance may occur from day to day even under highly controlled circumstances. When the unexpected is introduced, marked decline in performance may be seen because of the increased cognitive demand for flexibility in problem solving strategies (Savage and Wolcott, 1994; Ylvisaker and Savage, 1994; Blosser and Depompei, 1994).

Periods of vulnerability:

Situations, events, and circumstances requiring change and the application of new knowledge and skill can stress and tax the reserves of students with brain injuries. Common occurrences such as changes in schedules, classrooms or teachers may precipitate performance problems. Transitions from one developmental stage to another, movement from elementary to middle or high school, and episodes of illness or periods of medication adjustment may result in performance decline or the emergence of new frustrations and challenging behaviors.

Educational planning and intervention should identify, target and address major transitions and developmental milestones of high risk situations requiring focused attention. An understanding of normal growth and development, age related physical changes, nutrition, rest/exercise needs, and health/ safety concerns can guide interventions and aid in projecting potential areas of vulnerability. Table 2. lists key developmental issues and associated brain injury implications.

Educational planning and intervention should identify, target and address major transitions and developmental milestones of high risk situations requiring focused attention.

Table 2.

Growth/Developmental Issues and Potential Implications for Brain Injury

School/Age	Growth/Development Considerations	Potential Implications for Brain Injury
Pre-school age	■ Vision farsighted ■ Frequent snacks needed for high energy level ■ Keen sense of taste (color, flavor, texture important) ■ Likes finger-foods ■ Requires rest, naps ■ Immature understanding of danger ■ Common illnesses (ear infections, urinary tract infections, viral infections)	■ Visual disturbances may go undetected without routine exams ■ Fatigue, rest/exercise & nutrition needs must be monitored as alterations will affect performance ■ Decreased sensation, taste or loss of smell may impact on appetite ■ Decreased memory may impact on ability to learn safety
Elementary/ Middle School-Age	■ Permanent teeth emerge ■ Lymphoid tissue growth ■ Increased height/weight ■ Pre-pubescent vasomotor instability (increased perspiration, increased sebacious gland secretion) ■ Common illnesses (urinary tract infections, upper respiratory infections, sinus infections)	■ Oral hygiene and dental care is essential, particularly if on Dilantin. ■ Increased perspiration/sebacious gland secretion may be further enhanced by autonomic hyperactivity from injury. ■ Nutritional needs for ossification and bone growth need to be considered. ■ Illness may increase fatigue and affect ability to perform.
High School-Age	■ High growth spurt period ■ Skeletal growth more rapid than muscle (clumsiness) ■ Increased basal metabolic rate ■ Increased nutritional needs ■ Sexual development ■ Body image concern ■ Common illnesses (viral infections, sore throats) ■ Heart/lung slows and decreased oxygen available during activity (fatigue)	■ Poor coordination/motor control may increase existing clumsiness. ■ Increased metabolic rate may result in the need for increased nutrition. ■ Fatigue may affect performance. ■ Physical limitations or scars may affect a child's body image and self-concept. ■ The need for peer approval may increase vulnerability for impulsive substance abuse.

Pharmacology and behavior:

Medications may be needed to control seizures, relieve depression and anxiety, reduce spasticity, and manage challenging behaviors. Commonly used drugs include anticonvulsants, antidepressants, neuroleptics, psychostimulants, and antianxiety agents. Meticulous management is essential because many of these medications exert a cognitive blunting effect (Feeney, and Urbanczyk, 1992). The goal is to achieve the desired results without impairing cognition or introducing unwanted side effects. Dosage adjustments and periodic monitoring of drug levels are often required to achieve optimal results.

The school nurse and the student's physician can play a key role in medication management and serve as the primary resource for educators regarding drug actions, indications, contraindications, and potential side effects. Inservice training on the essential observations needed for the major drug categories can alert teachers to signs of potential toxicity or unwanted side effects. These are listed in Table 3.

Table 3.

Common Medications, Potential Side-effects and Nursing Considerations

Drug Class	Common Medications	Potential Side-effects and Nursing Considerations
Tricyclic Antidepressants	■ Amitriptyline (Elavil) ■ Imipramine (Tofranil)	■ Most frequent side-effects are sedation and restlessness, confusion, inability to concentrate, urinary retention, and anorexia. ■ Dosage must be highly individualized according to age, weight and response. ■ Monitor for changes in vision, gastro-intestinal disturbances, cough or sore throat, bruising and changes in baseline behaviors.
Anticonvulsants	■ Carbamazepine (Tegretol) ■ Phenytoin (Dilantin) ■ Phenobarbitol	■ Tegretol should be taken with meals and tablets should be protected from moisture. Photo sensitivity may occur (use sunscreen). ■ Tegretol may cause blood discrasias; frequent blood cell evaluation must be conducted. ■ Dilantin may cause gum hyperplasia and bleeding (oral hygiene essential) and acne may develop (good skin care). ■ Phenobarbital may cause drowsiness, supervise the child's play to avoid safety hazards, falls

Table 3.

Common Medications, Potential Side-effects and Nursing Considerations *(continued)*

Drug Class	Common Medications	Potential Side-effects and Nursing Considerations
Psychostimulants	■ Methylphenidate (Ritalin) ■ Pemoline (Cylert)	■ Monitor weight on individuals using Ritalin, as weight loss is common. ■ Ritalin may cause Stevens-Johnson Syndrome (monitor for skin rash, fever, joint pain). ■ Insomnia is common with Ritalin and Cylert. ■ Cylert and Ritalin should not be used in children under 6 years of age.
Neuroleptics	■ Haloperidol (Haldol) ■ Prochlorperazine (Compazine)	■ Haldol may cause extrapyramidal effects (monitor for dystonias, dyskinesia). ■ Haldol may turn urine dark pink or reddish-brown. ■ Haldol may cause menstrual irregularity, or false/positive pregnancy results; for adolescent males, may decrease libido and breast enlargement. ■ Compazine must be stored in amber colored bottles. ■ Monitor for increased restlessness or excitement.
Antianxiety Agents (Benzodiazepines)	■ Alprazolam (Xanax) ■ Chlorazepate (Tranxene) ■ Lorazepam (Ativan)	■ Common side-effects include fatigue, confusion, dizziness, lightheadedness, crying, and disorientation. ■ Potential gastro-intestinal side effects (increased appetite, n/v, weight loss/gain, bitter taste) may be decreased if drugs are given with or shortly after meals. ■ Drugs must be tapered and gradually withdrawn; do not abruptly discontinue administering the drug. ■ Vivid dreams may be experienced, as well as sleep disturbances.

The Third "R": Reintegration

The greatest challenges students face are returning to his/her home, school, work and community (BIA, 1994). Successes after rehabilitation or rapid recoveries after even severe brain injuries can be rapidly undone if the reintegration of the student is not handled carefully and consciously.

Home/school/work/community:

The ultimate goal for all students with acquired brain injuries is successful reintegration and full participation in home, school, work, and community life. The ultimate aim of people involved with assisting individuals with brain injuries is to provide the necessary environment, conditions, and interventions needed to assist them in achieving this goal. Considerable coordination and integration is required to assure that needed services are available and provided in an appropriate manner. Adequate preparation of the schools, families, teachers, peers, and students is mandatory for successful school reentry (Savage and Ylvisaker 1994; Blosser and DePompei, 1994, 1990; Savage and Carter, 1988).

Several steps must be taken to assure that gaps in service provision do not occur. Early communication between school staff and hospital/rehabilitation clinicians can strengthen the joint development of an the initial Individual Education Plan (IEP). The school nurse can assist with interpretation of medical and clinical information regarding the nature, circumstances and effects of the injury, recovery course, medications, and treatment approaches. Inservice training and educational materials can be provided on various relevant topics such as common manifestations of brain injury, psychosocial adaptation issues, and medications.

The school nurse can also assure that the educational team meets regularly, especially regarding ongoing medical issues, and that the intervals for scheduled meetings are appropriate to the student's needs. Criteria for introduction, reduction, and modification of goals, classroom accommodations, and program interventions need to be specified and periodically reviewed. The nurse can help with identifying student strengths and parental expectations and assure that these are included in the educational plan. Integrated services require collaboration and communication. Accomplishing this within the time constraints of a busy and oftentimes overburdened educational schedule calls for creativity and ingenuity. The nurse can help energize and support the team by providing the inspiration, perspective and knowledge necessary to keep the team focused and motivated.

Conclusion

Promotion of health and wellness is essential for the optimal recovery of students with brain injuries. Health care professionals, especially the school nurse and the child's physician, can provide a vital link between the hospital and school and serve as resource persons for teachers overwhelmed by the medical complexities of students with brain injuries. They are essential members of the team necessary to monitor the impact of the injury on the whole child as they continue to develop and recover over time. Health care professionals can also help families understand the medical needs of their child and support the family with related medical issues. Involvement of these professionals in all aspects of the student's recovery and reintegration back to home and school will help the student and their family achieve greater success. The major considerations the school nurse needs to understand are listed in Table 4.

Table 4.

Major Considerations For Recognition, Recovery, and Reintegration for Individuals with Brain Injury

Recognition

Brain Injury
■ Traumatic
■ Non-traumatic
■ Diffuse

Levels of Severity
■ Mild
■ Moderate
■ Severe

Brain Components
■ Brainstem
■ Midbrain
■ Cerebrum
■ Cerebellum

Common Effects
■ Cognitive
■ Behavioral
■ Physical/Health
■ Communicative

Recovery

Characteristics
■ "Gappy" performance
■ Problems show up later in development
■ Recovery occurs over time with periods of regression/progression

Growth/Development
■ Pre-school
■ School
■ Adolescent

Periods of Vulnerability
■ Changes in people, places, things
■ Developmental transitions
■ Times of illness and stress

Health Promotion
■ Nutrition
■ Rest/exercise
■ Safety
■ Medication

Reintegration

Home
■ Parents
■ Siblings
■ Friends
■ Extended family

School
■ Teachers
■ Peers
■ Classroom
■ Extra-curricular

Community
■ Leisure
■ Work
■ Play
■ Love and relationships

XI Educating School-age Children Who Sustain Brain Injuries: Issues, OSERS Programs, Ongoing Needs

MARTHA R. BRYAN, ED.D.

NOTE: This chapter was developed in the author's private capacity and does not reflect views of the U.S. Department of Education.

According to reports in the literature and from the Brain Injury Association, brain injury is the most frequent cause of disability and death in children and adolescents in the United States (Lehr, 1990; Brain Injury Association, 1993; HEATH Resource Center, 1988). Statistics of incidence among children must be interpreted as "ballpark figures," however, as there are variations in the definitions and in the reporting of data, and not all cases are reported. A recent epidemiological study (Kraus, 1993) reports that in the United States there are 137,500 new hospital admissions each year for brain injuries among children under 15 (Note that these data only include children who are hospitalized; some may be treated in the emergency room or by private physicians and released). Of these, 6% are reported as severe, 8% as moderate, and 86% as mild. Some 24,000 are returning to the community each year with health-related needs. Of the 110,000 with mild brain injury, most have good recovery but with some neurological sequelae. Other sources (e.g., Savage, 1990) show the largest group of people with brain injury to be in the 15 to 24 year-old-range, which would add a sizable number of youth over 15 who are in the public schools. According to Waaland (1990), since half of all injuries in the United States occur in individuals below the age of 25 and children are more likely to recover from brain injury than adults, the number of children and youth living with brain injury is substantial.

What are the educational issues and challenges surrounding the children and adolescents who sustain brain injuries? How has the Office of Special Education and Rehabilitative Services (OSERS) of the U.S. Department of Education responded? What specific programs has the Office of Special Education Programs (OSEP) funded? What are the continuing educational needs of school-aged children with brain injury?

Synopsis of Education Issues

During the past ten years, there has been an increasing recognition of the incidence and impact of brain injury by some segments of our society. Progressive changes in technology and the enhanced delivery of emergency and acute care services have increased the recovery rate of persons with brain injuries will come through. Unfortunately, the health care delivery and community support services available have not expanded accordingly to meet the increasing needs of this population.

What is the impact on the schools? According to Kalsbeek et al. (1980), one in five hundred school-age children will be hospitalized each year because of a brain injury and, by age 15, 3% of the student body will have sustained a brain injury. Because the effects of brain injury may persist for years, the cumulative number of children who are struggling in school with the residuals of injury to the brain is larger than 3%. Mira and Tyler (1991) further project that an average city district can expect 90 to 100 children a year to sustain brain injuries and require education. In a small rural area, three or four children may be injured annually. Even with these statistics, however, Mira and Tyler (1991) note that brain injury is regarded as a low-incidence problem in the schools, with many school administrators reporting no occurrences. Thus, brain injury becomes a significant challenge for the schools, beginning with increased awareness of its existence.

An injury occurs involving the brain (external or internal cause), and suddenly the learning world is dramatically changed. First, the student and family encounter the trauma — with physical injuries, emotional shock and complications, and cognitive difficulties. A myriad of limitations may result: speech; vision; hearing and other sensory impairments; headaches; lack of coordination; spasticity of muscles; paralysis of one or both sides; and seizure disorders. Psychosocial, behavioral, and emotional impairments may include: fatigue; mood swings; denial; self-centeredness; anxiety; depression; lowered self-esteem; restlessness; lack of motivation; inability to self-monitor; difficulty with emotional control; inability to cope; agitation; excessive laughing or crying; sexual dysfunction; and difficulty in relating to others. The resultant cognitive problems are likely to include short term and long term memory deficits; slowness of thinking; and impaired concentration, attention, perception, communication, reading, writing, planning, sequencing, and judgment abilities (Brain Injury Association, 1989).

Unlike adults, brain injury in children involves understanding two processes that are occurring simultaneously — the process of recovery/improvement from injury superimposed on the overall years, rapid development and learning are still occurring in that the connections between the two hemispheres of the brain and between areas of each hemisphere are becoming more efficient. The interconnections between primary, sensory/perceptual/motor and association areas increase the ease in learning such academically related activities as reading, spelling, writing, arithmetic, and reasoning. At this point, children are expected to learn in groups, engage in activities outside the home, and on some occasions be under the direction of adults other than their parents.

Brain injury can interfere with academic, emotional, and psychosocial functioning during this period. The effect of brain injury may be the most significant for children who have not yet mastered the basics of reading, writing, and mathematics prior to injury. Controlled processes that underline learning, such as attention, memory, and speed of information processing, have a direct impact on learning (Lehr and Savage, 1990).

The student who sustains a severe injury will participate in a rehabilitation program of variable length depending on the severity of the injury.

Most of the students sustain mild to moderate injuries which result in a variety of these impairments — some of which may not be reported to the schools. These students will likely re-enter school following brief medical treatment without a rehabilitation program. The student who sustains a severe injury will participate in a rehabilitation program of variable length depending on the severity of the injury. This program may include retraining in any of the above-described areas, including cognitive retraining.

Tucker and Colson (1992) describe recovery as a long, slow process that could be enhanced by attending school in a supportive environment with an appropriate educational schedule and plan in place before reentry. Students are frequently misclassified as individuals with learning disabilities or emotional disturbances. Savage (1993) further points out that often when the young child's brain is injured, more serious cognitive and emotional difficulties emerge as the brain matures. Soon after the injury, the child may appear "normal" but will encounter problems at a subsequent developmental stage when higher order cognitive skills are essential.

What are the student's needs expected to be, upon reentry into school? The literature (Begali, 1992; Lash, 1992; Martin, 1988) asserts that the emotional issues in the loss which has occurred for both the student and the family must be understood by the educator. As well, there may be some recognizable differences in the child's emotional responses as a result of the injury. Martin (1988, p. 464) states that "it is vitally important for educators and health professionals who work with children with brain injury to understand the nature of the family's experience and their special perspective." The family has experienced the loss and is participating in the rehabilitation process. The family members' partnership in the educational planning is vital as it includes their observations and involves them in carrying out the intensive learning activities.

In understanding the complexity of brain injury, the educator needs to be aware of the emotional, psychosocial, and cognitive issues. It is important to understand the nature of the injury and the process for regaining cognitive function, particularly the changes which occur within the first year post-injury. Frequent re-evaluations are especially important during the twelve months post-injury. The person with brain injury's inability to recognize his or her own loss should be appreciated. Since the functions of the brain develop over a period of time, it is important to know the stage of development the student is in at the time of injury and to observe the child for the onset of other subsequent difficulties in the future. The long-lasting effects of brain injury need to be understood. Also, the cognitive issues must be interpreted by a neuropsychological and psychoeducational assessment.

Since injured brain tissue cannot be restored, there is likely the need for learning compensatory strategies.

Not only must the student be evaluated in terms of what has been retained of what was learned, but also, as specifically as possible, how the student can best learn in the future. Since injured brain tissue cannot be restored, there is likely the need for learning compensatory strategies. Hence to facilitate learning, the educator and team of professionals need to understand the conceptual models and approaches to cognitive retraining. These include memory, organization, concentration, and sequencing. For the child whose brain is continuing to develop, it is helpful to understand the impairment within the context of developmental theory.

The effects of the brain injury may have implications for the child's educational program. Within the provisions of the Individuals with Disabilities Education Act (IDEA), the student with traumatic brain injury (TBI), along with other eligible students with disabilities, is entitled to special education and related services. The range of potential services begins with such minimal intervention as specialized consultation with the classroom teacher regarding the needs of a given student and moves to increasingly specialized and intensive services.

Gerring (1992) points out that it is often the tendency of the school system to initially provide the setting that appears to be the least structured and to then increase the intensity of services if the child demonstrates a lack of progress. For some children who have sustained a brain injury, Gerring suggests this may not be the best practice. For some individuals who have sustained a brain injury, it is best to provide increased structure and intervention at the initial reentry and gradually reduce the intensity of services as the needs of the student change. For these individuals, increased structure is reassuring and minimizing distractions will enhance the student's ability to absorb information, which may be accomplished in a regular classroom or in a special education arrangement. Each child, however, must be evaluated individually by an interdisciplinary team to determine the most appropriate level of structure and intensity of services.

History of OSERS Response

This chapter will later describe some of the projects supported by the Office of Special Education and Rehabilitative Services (OSERS) of the U.S. Department of Education which address the educational needs of children with brain injury. As an introduction, a brief history of the agency's involvement in brain injury issues follows.

An Interagency Task Force was established by the Secretary of the Department of Health and Human Services in 1988 to recommend solutions for meeting the needs of persons with brain injury. Subsequently, rehabilitation centers were funded by the Rehabilitation Services Administration (which will be described later in the chapter and listed in the Resources Section). Also, research and model demonstration projects (listed in the Resources Section) were supported by the National Institute on Disability and Rehabilitation Research.

In the summer of 1991, a Memorandum of Understanding (originally signed in 1985) was renewed between the Brain Injury Association, the Office of Special Education and Rehabilitative Services (including its components of the Office of Special Educations Programs, the Rehabilitation Services Administration, and the National Institute on Disability and Rehabilitation Research), the Council of State Administrators of Vocational Rehabilitation, and the National Association of State Directors of Special Education. The parties to this memorandum agree to cooperate in facilitating expanded research and improved delivery of education and rehabilitative services that will enhance opportunities for persons with disabilities caused by brain injury to achieve community reintegration and to receive social support for themselves and their families.

In 1991, traumatic brain injury was added as a category in the Rules and Regulations for the Education for the Handicapped Act (Public Law 99-457). This category was intended to promote both an understanding of and appropriate response to the diverse educational needs of the student, thereby discouraging mislabeling of the student with TBI. The definition included in the current Rules and Regulations (Federal Register, 57, 1992, p. 44802) for the current law, the Individuals with Disabilities Education Act (Public law 101-476) follows:

> "Traumatic Brain Injury" means an acquired injury to the brain caused by an external physical force, resulting in total or partial functional disability or psychosocial impairment, or both, that adversely affects a child's educational performance. The term applies to open or closed head injuries resulting in impairments in one or more areas, such as cognition; language; memory; attention; reasoning; abstract thinking; judgment; problem-solving; sensory, perceptual and motor abilities; psychosocial behavior; physical functions; information processing; and speech. The term does not apply to brain injuries that are congenital or degenerative, or brain injuries induced by birth trauma.

Students who sustain brain injuries from an internal cause, (e.g., aneurysm, stroke, anoxia, or tumor) can be eligible for services if their educational performance is adversely affected by the injury. However, they may be classified as having "other health impairment," "learning disability," or "multiple disability," although it is recognized that their educational and related services needs are similar to those who sustain a brain injury from an external force.

In 1991, the TBI category was entered into the data collection system for Part B (ages 6-21) of the Individuals with Disabilities Education Act. During the 1991-1992 school year, 330 children were reported as being served. For the 37 states which reported zeroes in this category, a possible explanation is that their State systems for data collection had not yet been converted to include the new category. Thus children with brain injury were included under "other health impaired" or other categories. Preliminary data for the 1992-1993 school year show dramatic increases in the numbers of identified students with brain injury who are receiving services with the total exceeding 3000.

OSERS Resources

National Institute on Disability and Rehabilitation Research, OSERS

The National Institute on Disability and Rehabilitation Research (NIDRR) has funded research and model demonstration projects in the rehabilitation of children and adults with brain injury since

1987. These projects (listed in Resources Section) are continuing to develop model system of the delivery of rehabilitation services for persons experiencing brain injury and their families. In addition to the directed research, projects related to TBI have been funded in other discretionary programs. These include both field initiated projects and Mary E. Switzer distinguished fellows' research.

Some of the discretionary projects also include issues of reentry into the educational system. For example, the booklet, "When Your Child Goes to School After An Injury" (Lash, 1992) was developed by a grant (award #H133B80009) funded by NIDRR. One of the fellowships (H133F20004) is conducting research on staff-family involvement. An innovative research project (H133C20085) is developing an assessment instrument to evaluate multiple intelligences in order to plan interdisciplinary interventions.

There are numerous resources being developed by the NIDRR-funded projects which address issues of the family, school reentry, and education for children who sustain brain injury.

Rehabilitation Services Administration, OSERS

In 1990, the Rehabilitation Services Administration funded four regional Head Injury Centers for four years with 15 million dollars appropriated by Congress. Two additional centers were funded in 1992 for a period of four years. These centers (included in the Resources Section at the end of this paper) are addressing the unique challenge and situation of brain injury by: developing new models of service delivery (i.e., to improve job placement and retention, to improve the employment opportunities for persons with brain injury); identifying and eliminating barriers to providing effective services; developing and implementing outreach programs to expand the knowledge and skills of personnel providing services to persons with brain injury; improving linkages among services and their providers to create models of integrated and coordinated care that are both comprehensive in scope and cost effective; improving linkages among services and their providers to create models of integrated and coordinated care that are both comprehensive in scope and cost effective; improving follow-up of people with brain injury to decrease secondary complications; strengthening the collaboration among survivors, their families and service providers; and improving and expanding brain injury prevention programs.

The centers include some focus on school reentry and education issues. For example, the booklet, "Guide Booklet on Traumatic Brain Injury in Children and Adolescents," (developed by and available from the Southwest Center) includes specific topics/issues related to accessing special education services and resources for integration. Additionally, "Head Injury: What Educators Need to Know" (developed by and available from the New York Center) is devoted to family issues, school reentry, assessment, program planning, and Individualized Educational Program (IEP) Development.

Office of Special Education Programs, OSERS

Three of the five divisions within OSERS have discretionary funding authority provided by IDEA. They are the Division of Personnel Preparation, the Division of Educational Services, and the Division of Innovation and Development. The individual program priorities offered by the three Divisions address research and development issues concerning the education of children with disabilities, including those with TBI, and training of personnel including teachers, related service personnel, parents and significant others.

Currently, there are two projects funded by the Division of Personnel Preparation (DPP) which address the educational needs of children with traumatic brain injury. In the Special Projects compe-

The individual program priorities offered by the three Divisions address research and development issues concerning the education of children with disabilities, including those with brain injury, and training of personnel including teachers, related service personnel, parents and significant others.

tition, the Preservice/Inservice Training Program in TBI (Cooley, 1991) is funded for five years to develop and implement a statewide model of preservice and inservice training for educators and parents who will serve students with traumatic brain injury. Specifically this project is: (a) developing and field testing inservice and preservice training modules including diagnostic and teaching methods, curricula materials, and resource linkages, (b) training a regional cadre of educational personnel to serve as inservice providers and consultants/resource persons for local education agency staff and parents; and (c) creating a system for on-going preservice and inservice training and dissemination of the TBI training model after the project has been completed.

Funded in the Low Incidence competition, the George Washington University (Kochhar and Krankowski, 1992) is developing a Master's level training program to prepare teachers and related services personnel to provide appropriate educational services for students with traumatic brain injury. The program offers specialization in brain injury with training emphasis in one of four areas: (1) assessment and diagnostics, (2) transition/interagency coordination, (3) educational planning and development, (4) cognitive remediation and technology. The curriculum content of the program enables participants to gain a comprehensive knowledge base and field experience for the appropriate delivery of educational services. In order to meet the needs of students with traumatic brain injury, participants will develop expertise in the following areas: academic and vocational assessment and programs, design of innovative curriculums and coordination of transition services. Course content integrates the roles of relevant agencies, begins with transition from hospital to school environments, and includes post-secondary planning, extended employment support, and transition to independent living.

The curriculum content of the program enables participants to gain a comprehensive knowledge base and field experience for the appropriate delivery of educational services.

The parent training and information centers supported by DPP grants assist parents of infants, toddlers, children, and youth. For students with brain injury, the parent centers provide information about educational issues, parent and student rights under Part B of IDEA, educational issues, parent and student rights under Part B of IDEA, assist parents with the development of IEP's for their children, and develop and disseminate relevant materials. Some of the Parent Training Centers have developed materials on children experiencing traumatic brain injuries. Traumatic brain injury advocacy centers may contact the parent center in their State to ensure that the center has adequate information about traumatic brain injury issues.

The Division of Educational Services (DES) is the second major component within OSEP which has discretionary grant authority. In the Transitions Branch of DES, two projects are currently funded which address the educational needs of youth with traumatic brain injury. One of the projects is awarded to the Massachusetts Statewide Head Injury Program (Kamen, 1992). The program is conducting a comprehensive follow-up study of people with traumatic brain injury who have transitioned from school into adult life. The resulting research will be used to design an exemplary transitional services model for people with traumatic brain injury aged 16-21 years. One hundred people with brain injury living and/or working in integrated community settings have been surveyed and their reports are being compared with a similar group of survivors working and living in non-integrated settings. Analysis of collected data will seek to identify variables that have contributed significantly to differences between successful and unsuccessful transitions. A model will then be developed describing the experiences, support services, and training that are most likely to result in transition to community settings. The model will then assist those concerned with the transition of people with traumatic brain injury in school restructuring, long-range planning, and personnel preparation.

In a second transitions project, (High, 1993), the Institute for Rehabilitation Research in Houston, Texas is conducting research designed to assess the effectiveness of selected strategies for providing transitional services to youth with disabilities, aged 16-21, who have sustained a moderate to severe insult to the brain. Approximately twenty youth with brain injury will be served in each project year. Through the use of a parent questionnaire, consultation with professionals, and provision of inservice training and technical assistance to agencies currently serving students with brain injury, staff will identify, develop, and test strategies for transitional case management; vocational training; and recreational, leisure, or social skills. Comprehensive follow-up studies will be conducted for the targeted population, results of which shall provide a foundation for the design of exemplary transitional services. The program will then develop and test the feasibility of cooperative efforts between education agencies and adult service agencies to provide comprehensive transitional services to the target population. Finally, staff will identify and test strategies for the transfer of assistive technology devices (communication, adaptive equipment, etc.) from the educational environment to employment and other community settings.

The program for Persons with Severe Disabilities of the Division of Educational Services has two projects for students with brain injury, both at the Teaching Research Division, Western Oregon State College. The first project (Sowers, 1991) is developing a model to improve the participation of students with traumatic brain injury, ages 13-21, in social and educational experiences. The project will develop an intervention package for children with traumatic brain injury. The package offers a range of options to students, including social skills training, and school- and community-based social network enhancement. The intervention components are based on techniques that have been empirically validated with students who have other disabilities, but will be modified to meet the needs associated specifically with brain injury. The package consists of both student-centered and environment-centered strategies.

The second project, a recently funded model inservice training project (Glang, 1993) at the Teaching Research Division, proposes to gain a holistic perspective of the issues associated with educating students with traumatic brain injury in general education settings. The researchers will evaluate the impact of an inservice training model aimed at coordination of regional services. Teams of professionals from each of seven regions throughout the state of Oregon will participate in developing the inclusion model of students with traumatic brain injury. The training is to be conducted in an intensive workshop format. The content will include information about brain injury, interventions to impact behavioral, academic, and social outcomes for students with brain injury, and consultation skills to facilitate collaboration among school personnel. Publication of the curricula and guides produced by the project is expected to have the widest impact.

The Division of Innovation and Development, the third major component of OSEP with discretionary authority, has one project (Guess, 1993) which has implications for infants and children who sustain brain injury. The study is systematically investigating changes in states during the first few months and years of life among 25 infants at high-risk for profound and severe disabilities. The research will identify variables and conditions that potentially impact the emergence of various state organization patterns. Findings from the project are expected to have additional implications for the assessment and treatment of behavioral changes and physical losses associated with traumatic brain injury.

In summary, these projects are beginning to explore problems and identify possible solutions to the multifaceted issues and ways of providing quality educational programs for students with brain injury. Three of the projects are developing better strategies for the delivery of services for children and youth with brain injury. The other three projects are addressing the needs for inservice and pre-service training of personnel who will provide services for students with brain injury. The research project could have implications for the assessment and treatment of persons with brain injury. It is expected that the projects will add to the body of available literature, from which to develop promising practices.

Ongoing Need

The literature describes efforts underway to improve the preparation of personnel and the delivery of services for students with brain injury. The Office of Special Education and Rehabilitative Services has joined with advocacy organizations to respond to the needs of persons with brain injury. Yet, at this point, there remain serious shortfalls in educational services.

As was previously indicated, the educational system is being asked to serve increasing numbers of children and youth who have sustained brain injury. These students often have long-term learning problems that include cognitive, behavior/psychosocial, sensory/motor, and language disorders. A lack of awareness and understanding of the unique characteristics and the educational needs of these students exists even among special education personnel.

Mira et al. (1992) states that school administrators are not clear on the responsibilities of rehabilitation agency personnel versus education staff for the child with brain injury. A survey conducted by Tyler and Mira (1988) revealed that most school principals in Kansas were not aware that children with brain injury are present in their schools. As a result of the lack of awareness many students are not provided with any rehabilitation services (Savage 1990). The data submitted to the Office of Special Education Programs by the State Departments of Special Education (1992) show that either systems for tracking are not in place or that assistance is needed with identifying the students. Some of the literature (Tyler and Mira, 1988; Mira and Tyler, 1991) suggests that school systems have not properly identified the students.

Once students with brain injury are identified, in order to receive an appropriate education, steps must be taken to provide training for both new and experienced teachers, related services personnel, and parents. Mira et al. (1992) notes that all school personnel need to be knowledgeable about traumatic brain injury. Inservice education is needed for regular and special education teachers, school psychologists, counselors, and social workers. The authors believe also that traumatic brain injury knowledge may soon be required for certification and recertification.

In a survey completed by Sowers (1991), teachers were asked to rate how prepared they were and how confident they felt in handling the social behaviors and peer relations of persons with traumatic brain injury. On a scale of 1-5 (1=not at all prepared; 5=very prepared), teachers mean responses were as follows: 3.0, facilitating peer relations: 2.1. Pretests administered by the Kansas special project (Cooley, 1992) indicate that some fifty percent of the special education teachers lack basic knowledge of the learning and psycho/social needs of students with traumatic brain injury. Another study completed at the University of Washington had similar findings (Reus, 1990). Kochhar (1992) identified areas in which special education programming has not effectively met the needs of stu-

The Office of Special Education and Rehabilitative Services has joined with advocacy organizations to respond to the needs of persons with brain injury. Yet, at this point, there remain serious shortfalls in educational services.

dents with brain injury are as follows: a) assessment, b) individualized education programming, c) placement, and d) teaching strategies.

While the training of personnel is a critical need, there is still little research available on prescriptive instructional methodology for students with brain injury (Miller, 1984). Due to the scarce research and the diversity of the group of learners, Martin (1988, p. 127) states that: "Practitioners are left to assume that sound teaching practices adapted to the learner and delivered with an appreciation for the possible sequelae of head injury have the same chance for success as they do when applied knowingly to other disabled learners." Some more recent literature (e.g., Ringle-Bartels and Story, 1993) describes use of a cognitive/developmental model which has evolved out of years of practice. Yet, few teaching techniques specific to traumatic brain injury have been empirically evaluated.

The long-lasting problems and erratic employment history of people who sustained brain injuries years ago suggests that both learning difficulties continue to exist. Mira, et al. (1992) report that both neurological and cognitive-behavioral effects of mild injury, including diffuse changes within the brain, memory and attention difficulties may persist. Lehr (1990) further states that little data are available about which interventions are most effective for reducing emotional and behavioral traumatic brain injury deficits.

The literature also suggests (Savage, 1988; Kamen, 1992; Gerring & Carney, 1992) that there is a need to improve the transition from the medical treatment team to the school. While it is believed that the transition should include a designated team to coordinate between the medical facility and the school, the involvement of families, and the preparation of school personnel, there are no empirical data that show which school reentry procedures are best.

The effects of brain injury are being recognized at earlier ages, and little research has been conducted on the developmental effects (Mira et al., 1992; Bagnato and Neisworth, 1989). What is known about the developmental effects (Allison, 1992; Savage, 1993) suggests that when an injury occurs in a young child, more serious learning and behavioral difficulties may appear as the brain develops. Some literature (Mira, Tucker, Tyler, 1992) indicates that a high percentage of brain injury in young children is not identified and some cases caused by abuse may not be reported. All of these factors substantiate the need for educators to be trained to recognize the appearance of injuries and to follow-up with the child with a known injury.

Since the highest incidence of brain injury occurs with the 15-24 age category, it is not surprising that most rehabilitation centers, including those funded by OSERS, are for young adults and not for school-age children. Consequently, may children do not have intense rehabilitation prior to school re-entry.

OSERS' response to the needs of children with brain injury has been significant. Similarly, the field has responded to the needs by developing information on appropriate interventions and implementing training programs to prepare personnel. Yet, there remain challenges for state and local education agencies and institutions of higher education to continue to develop strategies and to train teachers and other school personnel.

> While it is believed that the transition should include a designated team to coordinate between the medical facility and the school, the involvement of families, and the preparation of school personnel, there are no empirical data that show which school re-entry procedures are best.

126

Conclusions

The educational program for the child who has sustained a brain injury should address the unique needs of each student. It is recognized that families must be involved in the school re-entry process. Due to the multifaceted needs of the child with brain injury, there is a need for using an interdisciplinary approach to develop the program for the child. A number of training models are being developed and implemented. Some of the training and service delivery models are utilizing a cognitive/developmental approach which needs further validation. If proven effective, this model may have significant implications for other children with cognitive impairments. Each child with brain injury will have unique needs depending on the location and severity of the injury and the stage of the brain's development at the time of injury. In addition to neurological, occupational, physical therapy, and speech/language pathology assessments, neuro-psychological and psychoeducational assessments are needed to determine the cognitive and psychosocial strengths and weaknesses of the student. During the initial year following the injury, re-evaluation should be frequent, and evaluations should be conducted for long-term follow-up, especially with a child injured at an early age. Many rehabilitation programs are in operation and models are being developed for the transition from the hospital or rehabilitation center to the school. Results of a recent survey (Rehab Update, 1993) reaffirm that families and professionals agree that information about community organizations and resources is the greatest need of people with traumatic brain injury. Thus more effective strategies for the dissemination of existing knowledge and resources is needed.

> Each child with brain injury will have unique needs depending on the location and severity of the injury and the stage of the brain's development at the time of injury.

The needs for improvement in planning the best school re-entry and educational programming are apparent. Increased awareness is vital to ensure that the students with brain injury are properly identified. Many children with mild brain injuries are not being identified in special education; yet they are in need of support services in the regular classroom. Improved and expanded rehabilitation services for traumatic brain injury are needed, especially for younger children. More research on transition models (from rehabilitation to school), assessment techniques, interdisciplinary service delivery models, developmental aspects of injury, effective intervention techniques, long-term injury implications, and the efficacy of teaching techniques is critical. Inservice education with parents, educators, and school personnel is imperative. The inclusion of brain injury content in preservice education is also critical.

Although this chapter has only referenced some possible causes of brain injury, the schools may play a vital role in prevention programs through safety education as well as violence and abuse prevention programs. Advocacy groups, coordinated primarily by the Brain Injury Association and its state associations, are leaders in this effort. Models which they are developing (e.g., HeadSmart® Schools) could contribute to the nation's effort to reduce violence and substance abuse and thus prevent injuries. Prevention is the only real cure for brain injury.

References

Allison, M. (1992). The effects of neurologic injury on the maturing brain. Headlines. October/November, 22-24.

Bagnato, D.J. & Neisworth, J.T. (1989). Neurodevelopmental outcomes of early brain injury: a follow-up of fourteen case studies. Topics in Early Childhood Special Education. 9, 72-89.

Begali, V. (1992). Head injury in children and adolescents: A resource and review for schools and allied health professionals, 2nd edition. Brandon, VT: Clinical Psychology Press.

Bush, G.W. (1986). Coma to community. Paper presented at the Santa Clara Conference on Trauma Head Injury, Santa Clara, CA, April. Washington: National Head Injury Foundation.

Cooley, S.A. (1992). A statewide project to develop and implement training activities and materials for persons at the pre & inservice level work with traumatic brain injury students. Topeka, Kansas: State Board of Education. Special project (H024K10061).

DiScala, C., Osberg, J.S., Gans, B.M., et al. (1991). Children with traumatic head injury: morbidity: and post acute treatment. Architectural and Physical Medical Rehabilitation. 72, 662-666.

Gerring, J.P. & Carney, J.M. (1992). Head trauma: Strategies for educational reintegration, second edition. San Diego: Singular.

Glang, A. (1993). Model inservice training in traumatic brain injury. Eugene, Oregon: Oregon Research Institute, Inservice Training Model project (H086R30028).

Guess, D. (1993). Longitudinal assessment of emerging behavior state patterns among infants and children with severe and profound disabilities. Lawrence, KS: University of Kansas (H0223C30029).

The Head Injury Survivor on Campus: Issues and Resources. (1988) HEATH Resource Center, 1-10.

High, W. (1993). Transition of youth with TBI to integrated post secondary environments. Houston, TX: Brain Injury Research Center, Research project (H15830008).

Kalsbeek, W. D., McLaurin, R.L., Harris, B.S. & Miller, J.D. Lash, (1980). The national head injury and spinal cord survey: Major findings. Journal of Neurosurgery. 53, 519-531.

Kamen, D. (1992). Empirical analysis of the education experiences of young adult TBI survivors who live and work in integrated settings. Boston: Statewide Head Injury Program, Massachusetts Rehabilitation Commission, Model Demonstration Project (H158P20006)

Kehr, E. (1990). Incidence and etiology. In: Lehr, E., ed. Psychological management of traumatic brain injuries in children and adolescents. Rockville, MD: Aspen, 1-24.

Kraus, J.F. (1993). Epidemiology and impact of head injuries in children. Paper presented at Consequences of Traumatic Head Injury in children: Variability in Short and Long-term Outcomes, Bethesda, MD, November 18-19.

Kochhar, C. & Krankowski (1992). A professional training and development program for special educators with an emphasis in traumatic brain injury. George Washington University, Preservice training project (H029A20045).

Krankowski, T. (1993). Meeting the transition and postsecondary needs of students with traumatic brain injury. Special Topic Report # 1, Richmond: Regional Resource Trauma Center funded by NIDRR, Grant Award #H133B*0029.

Lash, M. (1992). When your child goes to school after an injury. Medford, MA: Tufts University.

Lehr, Ellen (1990). Community and social integration from a developmental perspective. In Jeffrey S. Kreutzer and Paul Wehman's (Eds.) Community reintegration following traumatic brain injury. Baltimore: Paul Brookes, 1990, 301-309.

Martin, D.A. (1992). Children and adolescents with traumatic brain injury: impact on the family. Journal of Learning Disabilities. 21, 464-469.

Miller, J.D. (1984). Assessing language production in children: Experimental procedures. Austin, Texas: PRO-ED.

Mira, M.P. & Tyler, J.S. (1991). Students with traumatic brain injury: Making the transition from hospital to school. Focus on Exceptional Children. 23, 1-11.

Mira, M.P., Tucker, B.F. & Tyler, J.S. (1992). Traumatic brain injury in children and adolescents: A sourcebook for teachers and other school personnel. Austin, TX: PRO.ED

National Head Injury Foundation (1989). Basic questions about head injury.

Office of special Education Programs. 1992 annual report to Congress, Table AA4.

Reus, B. (1990). School re-entry: Educational programs for students with brain injury. Presented at Brain Injury Update 1990: A Northwest Regional conference for Occupational Therapists and Physical Therapists. University of Washington, Seattle.

Ringle-Bartels, J. & Story, T.B. (1993). Treatment of acquired cognitive-communicative deficits in young children. Neurorehabilitation: An Interdisciplinary Journal. 3, 26-43.

Rosen, C.D. & Gerring, J.P. (1986). Head trauma: Educational reintegration. San Diego: College Hill.

Savage, R.C. (1988). Introduction to educational issues for students who have suffered traumatic brain injury. In R.C. Savage & G.F. Wolcott (Eds.), An educator's manual: What educators need to know about students with traumatic brain injury. Southborough, MA: National Head Injury Foundation.

Savage R.C. (1993). Children with traumatic brain injury. TBI Challenge. 1. 4-5.

Sowers, J.A. (1991). Enhancing social support and integration for students with traumatic brain injury. Eugene, Oregon: Oregon Research Institute, Model Demonstration project (H096D10008).

Tucker, B.F. & Colson, S.E. (1992). Traumatic brain injury: An overview of school re-entry. Intervention in School and Clinic. 27. 198-206.

Waaland, P.K. (1990). Family response to childhood brain injury. In: Kreutzer, J.S., Wehman, P., eds. Community integration following traumatic brain injury. Baltimore: Paul H. Brooks, 225-248.

Wolcott, G.F. & Lash, M. (1993). Parents and professionals identify research and information needs - Communication tops list. Rehab Update. Summer, 1-2.

Resources

Traumatic Brain Injury Centers - Funded by the Rehabilitation Services Administration, Office of Special Education and Rehabilitative Services, U.S. Department of Education

Eastern Regional TBI Center (1990–1994)
New York, New Jersey, Connecticut, Puerto Rico
Contact: Wayne A. Gordon, Ph.D. (212) 241-7917

Midwest Regional TBI Center (1990–1994)
Illinois, Indiana, Michigan, Minnesota, Ohio, Wisconsin
Contact: Don Olson, Ph.D. (312) 908-6179

Rocky Mountain Regional TBI Center (1990–1994)
Colorado, Montana, New Mexico, North Dakota, Wyoming, Utah
Contact: Sharon Mikrut, M.S.W. (303) 894-7556, Ext. 302

Southwest Regional TBI Center (1990–1994)
Arkansas, Louisiana, New Mexico, Oklahoma, Texas
Contact: L. Don Lehmukuhl, Ph.D. (713) 666-9550

Ohio Valley Regional TBI Center (1992–1996)
Indiana, Virginia, Ohio, West Virginia
Contact: John D. Corrigan, Ph.D. (614) 293-3830

Southeastern Regional TBI Center (1992–1996)
Alabama, Florida, Kentucky, North Carolina, South Carolina
Tennessee, Georgia, Mississippi
Contact: Thomas J. Boll, Ph.D. (205) 934-8723

Model Systems of Care — Funded by the National Institute on Disability and Rehabilitation Research, Office of Special Education and Rehabilitative Services, U.S. Department of Education

Wayne State University Medical Center 1987–1998
Detroit, Michigan
Contact: Mitchell Rosenthal (313) 745-9769

The Institute of Rehabilitation Research
Houston, Texas
Contact: Donald L. Lehmkuhl (713) 797-5731

Santa Clara Valley Medical Center
San Jose, California
Contact: Terry Englander, M.D. (408) 295-9896

Virginia Commonwealth University 1987–1998
Medical College of Virginia

Richmond, Virginia
Contact: Jerry Kreutzer (804) 786-0200

Research and Training Centers — Funded by the National Institute on Disability
and Rehabilitation Research

New York University Medical Center (Moderate Injury)
New York, New York 1987–1998
Contact: Martha Scotzin (212) 263-6189

The Medical College of Virginia 1988–1993
(Severe Injury/Coma Management)
Richmond, Virginia
Contact: Veronica Powell (804) 786-7290

University of Washington (Moderate Injury) 1988–1993
Seattle, Washington
Contact: Justus Lehmann (206) 543-6766

The Mount Sinai Medical Center 1993–1998
New York, New York
Contact: Wayne A. Gordon, Ph.D. (212) 241-7917

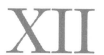

XII   Prevention –
What Can We Do In School?

MARY-GARRETT BODEL, M.ED, M.S.W.
EVE BERGER, M.A.

Brain Injury Prevention and Kids

What's the number one killer and disabler of youth in America? AIDS? Other infectious diseases? Food poisoning? Drugs?

In the United States, brain injury is the leading cause of death and disability among people under 24 years of age. A brain injury occurs every 15 seconds; every five minutes one of these people will die and another will be permanently disabled (Interagency Head Injury Task Force Reports, National Institute of Neurological Disorders and Stroke, National Institutes of Health, Bethesda, M.D.). Unlike a broken bone, a "broken" brain will never be the same again. A brain injury affects memory, speech and language, vision, the ability to walk or keep a stable body temperature, and even their personality or temperament.

While injuries are often considered acts of fate, like diseases, they can occur in highly predictable patterns and are often preventable. They are not "accidents." Injuries can be either unintentional or intentional. Unintentional injuries include automobile and traffic related mishaps, falls off of playground equipment, bikes, horses or out of windows; and sports injuries often acquired from contact sports, boxing, skiing and diving. Intentional injuries include assaults, gun shots, and child abuse. Children and adults often engage in these activities wihtout ever thinking of what "might" happen.

When we discuss the prevention of traumatic brain injuries we must include those children who have already sustained brain injuries as much, if not more than those in the mainstream. Children who have a brain injury as we have learned, may be less likely to have full use of all their motor skills, balance and judgement. Prevention for these children is even more important.

> People can lose memories, the ability to speak and write, vision, the ability to walk or keep a stable body temperature, and even their personality or temperament.

Motor Vehicles and Brain Injury

More than half of all brain injuries occur from motor vehicles and traffic incidents. These injuries happen to children as occupants in cars or as pedestrians. In a 30 mph automobile crash, a ten pound infant is thrust forward with the force of 200 pounds, and the 100 pound adult who is holding the child would crush it with a 3000 pound force (American Automobile Association, 1991). Proper use of seat belts and child safety seats have a proven history of preventing injuries for occupants of motor vehicles (American Automobile Association, 1991).

Child safety seats for infants and booster seats for young children should always be used whenever a child is a passenger in a vehicle. The seat should be securely anchored to the vehicle or it may become a launch pad in a crash. Child safety seats come in three sizes and are based on the weight of the child. An infant safety seat can hold infants weighing up to 20 pounds, a convertible safety seat will hold an infant weighing up to 40 pounds and booster seats will hold toddlers weighing 30 pounds and over. Children and teens should always be secured with safety belts, whether in the front or back seats of any motor vehicle. Belts should fit snugly around passenger's waist and lay flat across the shoulder.

As you interact with parents, please encourage them to always read the manufactures instructions that accompany the carseat and to follow the directions extremely carefully when installing the seat. Be sure that shoulder and lap straps are adjusted properly to hold the child in the seat if a crash occurs. Research on the effectiveness of child safety seats has found them to reduce fatal injury by 69% for infants and 47% for toddlers up to four years old (NHTSA, 1994).

Pedestrian injuries peak for children ages five to nine (Children's Safety Network, 1991). Children in this age bracket are at high risk for incurring an injury as a pedestrian because they are often developmentally unready to manage traffic, and parents routinely overestimate their children's abilities in this area (Frederick Rivara et al: Pediatrics, Vol. 88, 1991). Parents would laugh at the idea of giving a six-year-old "Gone with the Wind" to read, but saw no discrepancy in asking the same child to negotiate a familiar, but busy, intersection.

Children in this age bracket have one third the peripheral vision of adults. They also have difficulty judging speed and distance of moving vehicles, as well as determining the source of sounds. These perceptual skills are learned with practice as the child matures. Finally, children this age are short; they cannot see or be seen as well as an adult pedestrian, and they are often out on the streets without an adult.

Children have a single focus of concentration making it difficult for them to notice the sudden changes that occur with moving traffic.

A child's thinking at these ages is also not conducive to monitoring traffic. Children have a single focus of concentration, making it difficult for them to notice the sudden changes that occur with moving traffic. They haven't yet developed the adult's mental capacity to juggle several levels of thought simultaneously. Children tend to be self-centered. Little ones will run across the room with their eyes shut so they cannot be seen, and even eight- nine- and ten- year-old children believe if they can see the car, the car can surely see them. Children tend to be spontaneous and fanciful. Smaller children may think a car can see them with its headlights, and even nine-year-olds are not above darting into the street after a ball or frisbee.

Common child pedestrian injury scenarios include a child darting into street at mid-block or corner, a child entering the street from between parked vehicles, a vehicle turning into path of child pedestrian, a vehicle backing up into path of child pedestrian and a child entering or leaving school bus.

When working with children on the safety of crossing the street, stress the fact that not only do they need to watch for vehicles, but they must make themselves as visible as possible to drivers. Risk can be greatly reduced by not walking on roads at night, by walking on the side of the road facing traffic, and by wearing clothing that contrasts well with the surrounding environment.

One activity that you can do with your class is to introduce them to retroreflective tape. Set up a dark room in school with retroreflective tape on a few objects around the room. Take children to the room and have them try to see the items previously marked with tape. Discuss how much more visible items are with retroreflective tape on them. Ask students where they could wear the tape (hats, jackets, bookbags, etc.). Work with students to mark their outer clothing or bookbags with interesting designs and encourage them to leave the tape on their belongings.

When teaching safe pedestrian behaviors, you must help children to realize that they are not the only ones involved when they cross the street. Together with your class, create a cross walk in the school yard and have children act as different objects that can be present in any given situation (cars - parked and moving, people, trees, stop signs, etc.). Create a variety of situations that can occur and work through each one while teaching safe behaviors to the class.

Here are some safety pointers children should learn to prevent pedestrian mishaps:

■ Stop at edge of parked car, curb or vehicle

■ look LEFT-RIGHT-LEFT- for moving cars

■ cross only when clear and keep looking both ways

■ walk, never run or dash into street

■ look for signs that a car is about to begin moving (lights on, wheels turning)

■ always be alert

Falls and Brain Injury

Many brain injuries occur as the result of falls. Falling from windows, on stairs, off of playground equipment onto hard surfaces and off of bicycles can all result in brain injury.

Playground Equipment

Playgrounds are for children. Jungle gyms, sliding boards and swings allow children to develop coordination and practice skills, and they present age-appropriate challenges for children to master. But even with adequate supervision, falls do happen. Adequate surfacing under playground equipment can greatly reduce the occurrence of brain injuries sustained when children fall off of equipment.

The surface under climbing equipment should be able to absorb the shock of a falling child to reduce impact. The worst surfaces are asphalt and cement, closely followed by dirt, earth, or grass. Materials that are more appropriate are: wood mulch, wood chips, sand, gravel, and shredded tires. However, you do not want to increase one hazard while reducing another. Multi-colored rubber filler had to be replaced at one pre-school playground when the educators realized that the children were putting the bits in their mouths.

If your school has a playground with inappropriate surfaces, you should consider what steps are needed to change the surface. A group of concerned parents (PTA group) or contacting your Board of Education are often the best ways to achieve results.

When teaching playground safety to children, cooperation and sharing are always important behaviors to stress. Encourage walking, not running in the playground and to enforce taking turns when using equipment. Cooperative problem solving and conflict resolution are activities that can be used to help children learn to play together without conflict or fighting.

For further information on detailed specifications and how to improve the safety standards of your play ground you can contact the US Consumer Product Safety Commission, Washington, DC: 800-638-2772, and ask for their handbook for public playground safety

Falls from stairs and windows can also be prevented with some preparation. Stairwells should be well-lighted, level, and of appropriate height and width to avoid tripping. Slipping can be reduced by covering stairs with non-skid materials. Edges of handrails should be covered to avoid potential falls. Windows in schools are usually well-guarded, but make sure window guards are secure and that children cannot fit through them, but that they can be opened in the event of a fire. Sharp edges on desks and furniture can be covered with energy-absorbing padding.

Safety in the halls and stairs of schools should be taught much in the same way as playground and pedestrian safety. Halls and stairways, like intersections, are not a place to play. Again, walking should be stressed over running. Stay with your partner and walk together at the same pace. Create a game of safe hall and stair behavior and encourage children to always play the game when walking through school.

Bicycles

The most prevalent type of fall which results in brain injuries is from a bicycle. More than 600 children will die from bicycle injuries this year, most only a few blocks from home. A child is four times more likely to be seriously injured in a bicycle crash than to be kidnapped by a stranger. More children are killed and injured each year on bikes than on skateboards, roller skates, big wheels and scooters combined. (Brain Injury Association, 1993).

The majority of brain injuries sustained while bicycle riding occur among children ages ten to fourteen (Children's Safety Network, 1991). These children ride bicycles regularly, tend to be risk-takers, and deal with adult-level traffic situations without the proper training or equipment.

Bike helmets reduce the risk of brain injury by 85% and the risk of traumatic brain injury by 90%. A bike helmet costs about as much as one video game or five movie tickets. Only 5% of child cyclists currently use bike helmets (Children's Safety Network, 1991).

So how do we encourage children to wear helmets when bike riding? The answer may well be the two-pronged approach of education and legislation. A recent study comparing Howard County, Maryland which combined an educational campaign with helmet legislation, with Montgomery County, Maryland, which had an educational campaign but no legislation, indicated that helmet use more than tripled after helmet legislation was put into effect, following an intensive educational campaign. Andrew Dannenberg, M.D., the Johns Hopkins physician who led the study states, "such a campaign (educational) is not as effective unless it is combined with legislation." (Folkenberg, 1993).

Findings from Australia support Dannenberg's position. Australia is the first country to legislate the use of bike helmets nationwide and preliminary reports on the effectiveness of the measure are encouraging. In the Northern Territory, helmet usage rates jumped from 19% to 86% for commuters, from 26% to 71% among high school students and from 55% to 82% among primary school children. In Queensland a helmet usage rate of 82% was recorded among primary school children four months following legislation. "It is quite clear that helmet wearing rates have increased dramatically since mandation in every State and Territory for which data are available. (Injury Issues Monitor, p 3,4 1992)."

Another study which examines the effectiveness of bicycle helmets by examining data on casualties from Australia and Seattle, Washington also provides evidence of the benefit of legislation mandating helmet usage. (McDermott, et al, 1993).

However, as Dr. Norman McSwain, Jr. from Louisiana (McDermott et al, 1993) explains, "There are three subjects that are not compatible with polite conversation at a party, at a dinner table, or at a bar. The classic two are politics and religion; the third... is mandatory helmet legislation of any kind." People have a real love-hate relationship with the government about issues of public safety. It was evident with tobacco and alcohol warnings, safety belts and safety seat legislation, and now with the concept of bike helmet legislation.

Yet many states already have some form of helmet legislation, and the evidence is growing that the tide of public opinion is changing as parents and educators become more aware of the issues. In a recent nationwide telephone survey of parents, 73% favor mandatory bicycle helmet use for children age 14 and under and 79% want the government to help protect their children through more child safety laws (Campaign Update, January/February 1993). Findings from Australia also indicate that public attitudes were favorable, with 89% of the respondents indicating their support for the legislation. (Injury Issues Monitor, 1992).

Proponents of bike legislation urge mandatory helmet usage for all cyclists, because all cyclists are at risk for sustaining brain injuries, not just children, and such a law is easier to enforce. But Americans have been traditionally more willing to mandate safety rules for children, and children do sustain more brain injuries than any other segment of the population. Helmet laws for children are certainly a way to begin the process of behavior change. After all, how many adults do you know who finally began wearing a seat belt after they were asked to do so by their child?

Other thoughts on bicycle legislation include requiring that a helmet be part of the purchase of a child's bicycle (Folkenberg, 1993), and that bicyclists who ride in traffic be licensed like every other vehicle driver (Agran, et al. 1993). With licensure, young children would be less likely to be permitted to "play" in the streets on bicycles, and would be less likely to be riding in traffic when they are not developmentally ready to do so.

But perhaps the best reason to establish helmet legislation for children is so that when your child whines at you for the ninety-ninth time, "Why do I have to wear a helmet?", you can just answer, "It's the law, dear." End of discussion.

In regards to educational programs or methods to encourage helmet use and safe biking practices, the method is again, two-fold. Teaching both the necessity of wearing a bike helmet, and safe biking skills and behaviors is important.

A helmet is a means of protecting your head. Activities you can use to stress the importance of such protection may include using eggs or melons. Have children drop them from different heights. Discuss that the shell and rind are protection, but not enough protection when the object hits the floor. Use animals too, as an example. A turtle has a shell, a deer has antlers, a porcupine has needles. Why? They are all protective devices as is a helmet. These comparisons can help children understand how fragile their head and brain are and that it needs extra protection in certain situations.

When teaching about helmet usage, children should learn what type of helmet to wear and how to wear it correctly. Helmets should be ANSI or Snell approved. These two safety standards ensure that the helmet has been safety tested. Many helmets are available on the market that are not tested for safety. Make sure the helmet fits snugly and that the rider knows how to adjust the chin straps for a secure fit. The helmet should sit straight on the rider's head, not tilted back or forward. Children should be taught to wear a helmet every time they ride, even in their own driveway. Encourage parents to teach this simple lesson: no helmet - no bike.

The safest place to ride a bike is on special bike paths separated from motor vehicle traffic. Remember, a bicycle is not a toy, it is a vehicle. Teach children to follow the safety rules of the road:

Proponents of bike legislation urge mandatory helmet usage for all cyclists, because all cyclists are at risk for sustaining brain injuries, not just children, and such a law is easier to enforce.

■ ride with the flow of traffic (1 out of 5 bike collisions are caused by wrong way riders)
■ stop and look before riding out of a driveway
  (over 50% of child fatalities occur when kids ride without stopping and looking)
■ stop at all intersections (over 60% of child fatalities and injuries occur at intersections)
■ use proper hand signals
■ wear bright clothes, safety gear and reflectors if you must ride at night.

Many activities can be done in the school setting that encourage helmet wear and safe bicycling practices. Bike rodeos and skill tests are fun activities that can help children learn bike safety and be rewarded for using their new skills at the same time. Bike rodeos can be done in school gymnasiums or school yards. Teach children safety skills and then set up a riding course where they must follow the safety rules (like a driving test). When they finish the course they can receive a reward or certificate for a job well done, or they can re-do the course until they successfully complete it. For information on how to put on a bike rodeo in your school, contact your local Highway Traffic Safety Administration or Bike Helmet Safety Institute at 4649 2nd Street, South, Arlington, VA 22204 or Bicycle Federation of America at 1818 R St, NW, Washington, DC 20009.

> **It is just as important to follow safety rules when using these methods of transportation as when you are biking so be sure to teach your students to follow the rules.**

We are finally beginning to associate bikes and helmets together, but have yet to connect rollerskates, in-line skates and skateboards with helmets. The speed and sensation of flying gives kids a feeling of freedom as well as a means of sustaining injuries. The majority of people using this equipment (over 80%) do not use any protective gear at all. Bike helmets should be worn whenever using skateboards, in-line skates or rollerskates. Other protective gear that should also be used includes elbow, knee and shin pads. It is just as important to follow safety rules when using these methods of transportation as when you are biking so be sure to teach your students to follow the rules.

Other riding vehicles, like riding toys for small children, can be misused and cause brain injuries. Children two to four years of age are most often injured due to their level of curiosity yet their physical abilities are still developing. If these toys are available for the younger children in your school, consider these issues when determining who rides or where they will ride:
■ physical ability of the child
■ never let them stand on a toy meant for sitting
■ never let them coast down hills, they can gain too much speed
■ read all instructions to know how the toy should be operated
■ always supervise any child on a riding toy
■ keep toys and riders in an enclosed area, playground to make sure that they
  are not in danger from traffic.

Sports and Brain Injury

Professional and school organized sports, such as football, baseball, hockey, lacrosse and others, have rules and regulations about safety, illegal hitting, and helmet or protective gear use. Yet, when adults and children engage in these sports for fun, without the guidance of a league or organization, protective gear and helmets are rarely used. This can be dangerous for many reasons. The rules of the game may stay the same, so when tackling occurs in a casual game of football, 10 kids may still pile on top of one. Boys and girls will play together too, and due to size and strength differences, this can cause dangers as well.

When discussing contact sports with your students, encourage them to follow these rules:
- follow the rules like the professionals do - or change the rules to promote safety.
- wear protective head gear if the game calls for it
- designate a referee, so that rules are followed
- NEVER throw a ball, stick or piece of equipment at anyone.

Violence and Brain Injury

The United States is the most violent country in the world that is not at war. Many of our movies, books, and advertisements reinforce violent behavior, and our acceptance of it. Violence is rapidly becoming recognized as a major public health problem, and as such needs to be addressed through legislation and education. More than 160,000 children are seriously injured or impaired annually as the result of violence (BIA, 1993).

Child Abuse

The number of children who are physically abused and suffer head and neck injuries ranges from 50-60%. Seventy percent of children with acute brain trauma are victims of Shaken Infant Syndrome. (Brain Injury Association: Head Injury Resulting from Child Abuse, 1993). Babies and small children have large heads and weak neck muscles. In addition, the brain of an infant or small child is proportionately smaller than an adult's brain, and their skull is soft and pliable. When a child is shaken, the head whips back and forth and the brain slams against the inside of the skull. Shaking an infant can cause: blindness, deafness, paralysis, developmental disabilities, epilepsy, cerebral palsy, and death.

The social learning about how to respond to the world and solve problems that the same child will learn as he/she grows is equally destructive.

"Typically, a child's caretaker becomes frustrated - perhaps by the inconsolable crying of a colicky baby - and loses control. Grasping the child with thumbs on the sternum and fingers around the ribs and back, the caretaker shakes the child violently against the crib mattress" (Schroeder, September/October 1993). The resulting damage to the developing brain can be devastating. The social learning about how to respond to the world and solve problems that the same child will learn as she grows is equally destructive. However, if parents can be taught alternatives to violent discipline and how to interact with their child in a nurturing way, a great deal of damage can be corrected.

"The brain is very resilient and maintains an even course in the face of the most outrageous experiences. That is why children born in conditions of poverty and violence can still grow up normally, if the bad experiences are neutralized by a caring adult" (Kotulak, p12, August 1993).

In today's world, where there are so many teenaged parents and so many single parents the stress and frustrations of dealing with raising a child can be overwhelming. As educators we must take the responsibility to be on the look out for situations that are likely to result in the abuse of a child and take steps to prevent them.

If your school does not have parenting classes or parental discussion/support groups, you might consider starting them. Meanwhile you can stress the following to the parents in your class:

Shaking a baby is not discipline, it is child abuse.
Never shake an infant or small child.
IF YOU ARE ANGRY - DO NOT TOUCH THE BABY!

Instead: Shake a rug.
Take ten deep breaths.
Put the child in his or her crib.
Leave the room. Close the door.
Call a friend or neighbor.
Play loud music.
Take a shower.
Sit and relax for ten minutes.
Exercise.
Take a walk.

The violence epidemic is reflected in our statistics on injuries.

For further information about what you and your school can do to help prevent child abuse you can contact: The National Committee to Prevent Child Abuse, 200 State Road, South Deerfield, MA 01373-0200, Telephone: 800-835-2671.

Violence and Schools

Approximately one of every five high school students now carries a firearm, knife, razor, club, or other weapon on a regular basis, and many of them carry these weapons to school (Riley, 1993).

Violence appears in our society in many forms: homicide, assault, child abuse, child sexual assault, spousal violence, sexual assault, peer violence, and elder abuse. The violence epidemic is reflected in our statistics on injuries. A recent estimate puts intentional injuries, those created through acts of violence, at 50,000, roughly 1/3 of all injuries sustained in this country (Rosenberg, 1992). In certain areas in the country, and for certain segments of the population, the statistics are more sobering still.

"Certain factors increase the risk of violence. These include: racism, sexism, poverty, youth gangs, domestic violence, access to firearms, inadequate parenting, violent entertainment, child abuse, neglect, and the use of alcohol or other drugs" (Massachusetts Adolescent Violence Prevention Project, in Isaacs, 1992).

The causes of violence are complex so the solutions to violence must be comprehensive. Larry Cohen, director of the Prevention Program at the Contra Costa County Health Services Department, states, "This new solution suggests that the government must focus on violence as a public health issue, key organizations must work cooperatively, and prevention work must be based in local neighborhoods and schools" (Isaacs, 1992).

The Brain Injury Association concurs, and is working to be part of the solution by including violence prevention as part of the HeadSmart Schools head injury prevention program. Colman McCarthy, the founder and director of the Center for Teaching Peace states:

"Courses on nonviolence should begin in kindergarten and first grade, and continue through elementary school, junior high, and senior high school." In this way, we can begin to teach peace.

The HeadSmart Schools Program addresses violence by promoting the teaching of conflict resolution and cooperative problem solving as part of the regular school curriculum. These techniques can be used to help children learn to evaluate their own behavior, communicate with their peers and focus on finding solutions rather than fixing blame.

Learning to cooperate with other people in order to reach a goal is probably one of the most vital skills we need to live in our society today. The key is communication, and real communication is expressing what you believe and feel, and listening to what the other person believes and feels. Cooperation requires a willingness to put forth ideas for the group to try, and to try someone else's ideas as well. Children can build these skills while working on age appropriate puzzles, or tasks, that can only be solved by the group talking and working together.

Cooperative problem solving is a way to build communication and interpersonal skills while working in a group situation. Conflict resolution is a technique for managing a conflict once it has occurred. "Nobody practices negotiation because we have not been taught to negotiate. We practice conflict. It is the typical American way. When we want to solve a problem, we go to court" (Scherer, 1992, p.15).

Schools are faced daily with the need to manage conflict constructively. Traditionally, the adult resolves the conflict by imposing a solution or disciplining the students, which allows adults to become skillful at controlling students, but does not empower students to learn the procedures, skills and attitudes required to resolve conflicts constructively, so that they can regulate their behavior without an external monitor around (Johnson, et al. 1992).

Negotiation, or conflict resolution, can be taught, however, and many schools are teaching this process as a means to improve discipline and address the issue of violence in our schools. One teacher reports, "I have faith in the process of getting students to talk with one another. It's the only method I have seen work" (Scherer, 1992, p 15).

> Conflict resolution is a technique for managing a conflict once it has occurred. "Nobody practices negotiation because we haven't been taught to negotiate."

Steps to learning the techniques of cooperative problem solving and conflict resolution can be summarized as follows:

Cooperative Problem Solving

1. Own your feelings.
2. Trust your partners.
3. Communicate your ideas and feelings.
4. Listen to your partners.
5. Cooperate to work towards a solution.

Conflict Resolution

1. Tell your side. Use "I" statements.
2. Listen to the other person. Do not interrupt.
3. Repeat what the other person has said and ask what the other person wants you to do.
4. Tell what you want.
5. Generate two or three possible solutions.
6. Choose a solution.

Violence at Home

Violent behavior is cyclical. Children who experience violence as a way to communicate and solve problems will resort to violence as adults, teaching their children to do the same. Violence is learned behavior; alternatives to violence can be learned as well.

Parents can be proactive about violence reduction by becoming a role model, using non-violent discipline, letting children see adults having a respectful difference of opinion, refraining from celebrating violence in sports, and talking and listening to your children.

It is also important to resist media manipulation. Think about the things you view as entertainment, and what that communicates about the level of violence acceptance in your personal life-style. A movie ticket is a vote. What types of movies do you support?

Television networks live on advertising. What toys have you been buying that promote violence? Refuse to be "de-sensitized" to violence! If something offends you, say so. Violence is not funny, or sexy, or exciting. And finally, remember that you can always turn off the television.

Conclusion

The vast majority of brain injuries can be prevented, and at the present time, prevention is the only cure.

Most Americans are not used to thinking about their heads and brains, as vulnerable parts of the body. We are cautioned against fats to protect our heart, alcohol to protect our liver and sugar to protect our teeth, but the truth is the need to protect the head is tantamount. The vast majority of brain injuries can be prevented, and at the present time, prevention is the only cure.

"Prevention must be a part of health care, especially for children. Wellness and prevention must be woven into the rest of the school curriculum so that our children gain respect for their own bodies" (Surgeon General: C. Everett Koop, Healthy Kids Conference, 1992).

References

Agran, Phyllis, MD, MPH and Diane G. Winn, RN MPH, "The Bicycle: A Developmental Toy Versus a Vehicle," Pediatrics, Vol. 91, No. 4, April, 1993.

American Automobile Association, 1991 "Fragile, transport safely, a guide to child safety seats." Stock #3400.

Campaign Update, National Safe Kids Campaign, Vol. 6, No. 1. January/February 1993.

Children's Safety Network, A Data Book of Child and Adolescent Injury. Washington, DC: National Center for Education in Maternal and Child Health, @ 1991.

Folkenberg, Judy, "Legislation succeeds in encouraging use of bicycle helmets." NIH Healthline: Consumer health information from the National Institutes of Health. Bethesda, MD. 1993.

Injury Issues Monitor, Australia Institute of Health and Welfare, No. 1, December 1992.

Isaacs, M.R., Violence, the Impact of Community Violence on African American Children and Families, Arlington, VA. National Center for Education in Maternal and Child Health @ 1992.

Johnson, David, et al , "Teaching Students to be Peer Mediators," Educational Leadership, Association for Supervision and Curriculum Development, September, 1992, pp 10-13.

Kahane, C.J., "Correlation of NCAP Performance with Fatality Risk in Actual Head-On Collisions", National Highway Traffic Safety Administration, 1994.

Kotulak, Ronald "Casting new light on the brain," Washington Post, Health, August 31, 1993.

McDermott, Frank M.D. et al, "The effectiveness of bicyclist helmets: A study of 1710 casualties."

The Journal of Trauma, Vol. 34, No. 6, June 1993.

National Head Injury Foundation, "Pediatric Bicycle Injuries," Fact Sheet. 1993.

National Head Injury Foundation, "Head Injury Resulting from Child Abuse," Fact Sheet, 1993.

Riley, Richard, "Safeguarding our youth: violence prevention for our nation's children," United States Department of Education, Washington, DC. July 20, 1993.

Rivara, Frederick, et al "Prevention of pedestrian injuries to children: effectiveness of a school training program." Pediatrics. Vol 88.,October, pp 770 - 775, @ 1991.

Rosenberg, M. "Injury Control: Meeting the Challenge," Arch. Phys. Med. Rehabilitation, December, 1992, vol. 73.

Scherer, Marge., "Solving Conflicts - Not Just For Children," Educational Leadership, Association for Supervision and Curriculum Development, September 1992, pp 14-18.

Schroeder, Heather, MSJ, "Cerebral trauma," Headlines, September/October 1993.

Glossary

Abstract Thinking

Being able to apply abstract concepts to new situations and surroundings.

Acalculia

The inability to perform simple problems of arithmetic.

Acute Rehabilitation

Primary emphasis is on the early phase of rehabilitation which usually begins Program as the person is medically stable. The program is designed to be comprehensive and based in a medical facility with a typical length of stay of 2-3 months. Treatment is provided by an identifiable team in a designated unit.

ADL

Activities of Daily Living. Routine activities carried out for personal hygiene and health (including bathing, dressing, feeding) and for operating a household.

Affective Disorders

Mental illnesses characterized mainly by abnormalities in mood. The two principal categories are mania and depression.

Agnosia

Failure to recognize familiar objects although the sensory mechanism is intact. May occur for any sensory modality.

Agraphia

Inability to express thoughts in writing.

Alexia

Inability to read.

Anomia

Inability to recall names of objects. Persons with this problem often can speak fluently but have to use other words to describe familiar objects.

Anosmia

Loss of the sense of smell.

Anoxia

A lack of oxygen. Cells of the brain need oxygen to stay alive. When blood flow to the brain is reduced or when oxygen in the blood is too low, brain cells are damaged.

Anterograde Amnesia

Inability to consolidate information about ongoing events. Difficulty with new learning.

Aphasia

Loss of the ability to express oneself and/or to understand language. Caused by damage to brain cells rather than deficits in speech or hearing organs.

Aphemia

The isolated loss of the ability to articulate words without loss of the ability to write or comprehend spoken language.

Apraxia

Inability to carry out a complex or skilled movement not due to paralysis, sensory changes, or deficiencies in understanding.

Art Therapy

Use of art techniques such as painting, crafts and group activities to develop motor skills, perceptual abilities and self-esteem.

Associated Reaction

A non-purposeful movement that accompanies another movement (e.g., the arm may bend involuntarily when a person yawns).

Astereognosia

Inability to recognize things by touch.

Ataxia

A problem of muscle coordination not due to apraxia, weakness, rigidity, spasticity or sensory loss. Caused by a lesion of the cerebellum or basal ganglia. Can interfere with a person's ability to walk, talk, eat, and to perform other self care tasks.

Attention, Alternating

The ability to move attention appropriately from one area to another. It requires directional control, as well as capacity.

Attention/ Concentration

The ability to focus on a given task or set of stimuli for an appropriate period of time.

Attention/Concentration, Arousal

The ability to respond consistently tosensory stimulation by eye opening, localizing, and tracking with head or eye movement. To assess level of arousal one might determine if the person brushes away pinching fingers; or, if the eyes or head turns to a variety of sensory stimuli.

Attention/Concentration, Distractibility

Refers to the inability to sustain attention because of competing internal or external stimuli. Typically, the individual has decreased ability to inhibit competing responses. For example, a person who is restrained may focus more on his arm restraint than on a task presented by a therapist; a person asked to complete arithmetic problems may focus more on construction work taking place outside.

Augmentative and Alternative Communication

Use of forms of communication other than speaking, such as: sign language, "yes, no" signals, gestures, picture board, and computerized speech systems to compensate (either temporarily or permanently) for severe expressive communication disorders.

Automatic Speech

Words said without much thinking on the part of the speaker. These may include songs, numbers, and social communication; or, can be items previously learned through memorization. Spontaneous swearing by individuals who did not do so before their injury is another example.

Bilateral

Pertaining to both right and left sides.

Biofeedback

A process in which information not ordinarily perceived (such as heart rate, skin temperature or electrical activity of muscles) is recorded from a person and then relayed back instantaneously as a signal so that the individual becomes aware of any alteration in the recorded activity.

Brain Death

A state in which all functions of the brain (cortical, subcortical, and brainstem) are permanently lost.

Brain Injury

Damage to the brain that results in impairments in one or more functions, including: arousal, attention, language, memory, reasoning, abstract thinking, judgment, problem-solving, sensory abilities, perceptual abilities, motor abilities, psychosocial behavior, information processing and speech. The damage may be caused by external physical force, insufficient blood supply, toxic substances, malignancy, disease producing organisms, congenial disorders, birth trauma or degenerative processes.

Brain Injury, Acquired

The implication of this term is that the individual experienced normal growth and development from conception through birth, until sustaining an insult to the brain which resulted in impairment of brain function.

Brain Injury, Closed

Occurs when the head accelerates and rapidly decelerates or collides with another object (for example the windshield of a car) and brain tissue is damaged, not by the presence of a foreign object within the brain, but by violent smashing, stretching, and twisting, of brain tissue. Closed brain injuries typically cause diffuse tissue damage that results in disabilities which are generalized and highly variable.

Brain Injury, Mild

A mild traumatic brain injury is a traumatically-induced physiological disruption of brain function, as manifested by at least one of the following: 1) any period of loss of consciousness, 2) any loss of memory for events immediately before or after the injury, 3) any alteration in mental state at the time of the injury (e.g. feeling dazed, disoriented, or confused), 4) focal neurological deficit(s) which may or may not be transient; but where the severity of the injury does not exceed the following: a) loss of consciousness of approximately 30 minutes or less; b) after 30 minutes, an initial Glasgow Coma Scale score of 13-15; c) Post traumatic amnesia not greater than 24 hours.

Brain Injury, Moderate

A Glasgow Coma Scale score of 9 to 12 during the first 24 hours post injury.

Brain Injury, Penetrating

Occurs when an object (for example a bullet or an ice pick) fractures the skull, enters the brain and rips the soft brain tissue in its path. Penetrating injuries tend to damage relatively localized areas of the brain which result in fairly discrete and predictable disabilities.

Brain Injury, Severe

Severe injury is one that produces at least 6 hours of coma; Glasgow Coma Scale score of 8 or less within the first 24 hours.

Brain Injury, Traumatic

Damage to living brain tissue caused by an external, mechanical force. It is usually characterized by a period of altered consciousness (amnesia or coma) that can be very brief (minutes) or very long (months/indefinitely). Orthopedic, visual, aural, neurologic, perceptive, cognitive, or emotional impairments may result. The term does not include brain injuries that are caused by insufficient blood supply, toxic substances, malignancy, disease producing organisms, congenial disorders, birth trauma or degenerative processes.

Brainstem

The lower extension of the brain where it connects to the spinal cord. Neurological functions located in the brainstem include those necessary for survival (breathing, heart rate) and for arousal (being awake and alert).

Case Management

Facilitating access to relevant rehabilitation and support programs, and coordination of the delivery of services. This role may involve liaison with various professionals and agencies, advocating on behalf of the person and arranging for purchase of services where no appropriate programs are available.

Cerebellum

The portion of the brain (located at the back) which helps coordinate movement. Damage may result in ataxia.

Circumlocution

Use of other words to describe a specific word or idea which cannot be remembered.

Closed Head Injury

See Brain Injury, Closed.

Congenital Disability

A disability that has existed since birth but is not necessarily hereditary. The term birth defect is less desirable.

Cognitive Impairment

Difficulty with one or more of the basic functions of the brain; perception, memory, attentional abilities, and reasoning skills.

Cognitive Rehabilitation

Therapy programs which aid persons in managing specific problems in perception, memory, thinking and problem-solving. Skills are practiced and strategies are taught to help improve function and/or compensate for remaining deficits.

Coma

A state of unconsciousness from which a person cannot be aroused, even by powerful stimulation; lack of any response. Eyes are typically closed, there are no sleep/wake cycles. True coma does not last more than four weeks. Glasgow Coma Scale score of 8 or less.

Coma Vigil (See Persistent Vegetative State)

Communicative Disorder

An impairment in the ability to 1) receive and/or process a symbol system, 2) represent concepts or symbol systems, an d/or 3) transmit and use symbol systems. The impairment maybe observed in disorders of hearing, language, and/or speech processes.

Community Alternatives

Agencies, outside an institutional setting, which provide care, support, and/or services to persons with disabilities.

Community - Based Programs

Programs which are located in a community environment, as opposed to an institutional setting.

Community Skills

Those abilities needed to function independently in the community. They may include: telephone skills, money management, pedestrian skills, use of public transportation, meal planning and cooking.

Concrete Thinking

A style of thinking in which the individual sees each situation as unique and is unable to generalize from the similarities between situations. Language and perceptions are interpreted literally so that a proverb such as "a stitch in time saves nine" cannot be readily grasped.

Concussion

The common result of a blow to the head or sudden deceleration usually causing an altered mental state, either temporary or prolonged. Physiologic and/or anatomic disruption of connections between some nerve cells in the brain may occur. Often used by the public to refer to a brief loss of consciousness.

Confabulation

Verbalizations about people, places, and events with no basis in reality. The person appears to "fill in" gaps in memory with plausible facts.

Convergence

Movement of two eyeballs inward to focus on an object moved closer. The nearer the object, the greater is the degree of convergence necessary to maintain single vision.

Core Therapies

Basic therapy services provided by professionals on a rehabilitation unit. Usually refers to nursing, physical therapy, occupational therapy, speech-language pathology, neuropsychology, social work and therapeutic recreation.

Dance/Movement

The use of movement to music as a Therapy process which enhances, facilitates and integrates physical, cognitive and psychosocial function.

Deaf

Deafness refers to a profound degree of hearing loss that prevents understanding speech through the ear. Hearing impaired is the generic term preferred by some individuals to refer to any degree of hearing loss - from mild to profound. It includes both hard of hearing and deaf. Hard of hearing refers to a mild to moderate hearing loss that may or may not be corrected with amplification.

Developmental Disability

Any mental and/or physical disability that has an onset before age 22 and may continue indefinitely. It can limit major life activities. Individuals with mental retardation, cerebral palsy, autism, epilepsy (and other seizure disorders), sensory impairments, congenital disabilities, traumatic brain injury, or conditions caused by disease (e.g. polio, muscular dystrophy) may be considered developmentally disabled.

Diaschisis

A theoretical state following brain injury in which healthy areas connected to the damaged area show a temporary loss of function.

Discrimination, Auditory

The ability to differentiate and recognize sounds. This involves distinguishing between words, noises, and sounds that might be similar. A person with poor auditory discrimination might answer the phone in his room although the actual ringing came from an alarm clock.

Discrimination, Tactile

The ability to identify and distinguish between objects and stimuli solely through touch. This involves the ability to ascertain shape, size, and texture. For example, a person with impaired tactile discrimination might not be able to distinguish between a quarter and a dime in their pocket.

Discrimination, Visual

Involves the differentiation of items using sight. An individual with impaired visual discrimination may not be able to distinguish between a red and green light while driving or may have difficulty distinguishing between the letter "E" and the letter "F".

Doll's Eye Maneuver

The eyes appear to move in the direction opposite to the motion of the head, when the head is gently rotated.

Dysarthria

Difficulty in forming words or speaking them because of weakness of muscles used in speaking. Speech is characterized by slurred, imprecise articulation. Tongue movements are usually labored and the rate of speaking may be very slow. Voice quality may be abnormal, usually excessively nasal; volume may be weak; drooling may occur. Dysarthria may accompany aphasia or occur alone.

Echolalia

Imitation of sounds or words without comprehension. Is a normal stage of language development in infants, but is abnormal in adults.

Emotional Lability

Exhibiting rapid and drastic changes in emotional state (laughing, crying, anger) inappropriately without apparent reason.

Encephalography

Non-invasive use of ultrasound waves to record echoes from brain tissue. Used to detect hematoma, tumor, or ventricle problems.

Equilibrium

Normal balance reactions and postures.

Error Recognition

Refers to an individual's awareness that a response is incorrect for a task. The person may simply state, for example, "I know this is wrong", or show a confused, quizzical look after making an inappropriate response.

Executive Functions

Planning, prioritizing, sequencing, self- monitoring, self-correcting, inhibiting, initiating, controlling or altering behavior. Also referred to as "higher level functions."

Figure-Ground

The differentiation between the foreground and the background of a scene; this refers to all sensory systems, including vision, hearing, touch.

Fixation, Visual

A pause of the line of sight on something of interest in the visual world.

Fluently

Effortlessly smooth and rapid speech.

Focal

Restricted to one region (as opposed to diffuse).

Focus, Eye

Can imply: 1) convergence of the two eyes, 2) accommodation of the lenses of the two eyes, 3) tracking something by moving the eyes, 4) attending to something. Because the term has several meanings its use should perhaps be avoided.

Frontal Lobe

Front part of the brain; involved in planning, organizing, problem solving, selective attention, personality and a variety of "higher cognitive functions.

Glasgow Coma Scale

A standardized system used to assess the degree of brain impairment and to identify the seriousness of injury in relation to outcome. The system involves three determinants: eye opening, verbal responses and motor response - all of which are evaluated independently according to a numerical value that indicates the level of consciousness and degree of dysfunction. Scores run from a high of 15 to a low of 3. Persons are considered to have experienced a "mild" brain injury when their score is 13 to 15. A score of 9 to 12 is considered to reflect a "moderate" brain injury and a score of 8 or less reflects a "severe" brain injury.

Glasgow Outcome Scale

A system for classifying the outcome of persons who survive. The categories range from "Good Recovery" in which the person appears to regain the pre-injury level of social and career activity (even if there are some minor residual abnormal neurological signs); "Moderate Disability" in which the person does not regain the former level of activity but is completely independent with respect to the activities of daily life; "Severe Disability" is defined as a state wherein the conscious, communicating person is still dependent on the help of others. The original scale had five outcome categories, the newest scale has eight outcome categories. This scale relates to functional independence and not residual deficits.

Handicap

Describes a condition or barrier imposed by society, the environment, or by one's own self that limits or prevents the fulfillment of a role that is normal, depending on age, sex, and social and cultural factors, for the individual. Handicap can be used when citing laws and situations but should not be used to describe a disability. Not a synonym for disability.

Head Injury

Refers to an injury of the head and/or brain, including lacerations and contusions of the head, scalp and/or forehead. See Brain Injury.

Hemianopsia/Hemianopia

Visual field cut. Blindness for one half of the field of vision. This is not the right or left eye, but the right or left half of vision in each eye.

High Level Thought Processes

Includes conversion thinking, deductive and inductive reasoning, divergent thinking, and high level problem-solving, including comprehension of a problem, formulation of several alternative solutions based on past experiences or long-term memory, generation of a solution and evaluation of a solution. This differs from organization in that high level thought processes involve the use of multiple strategies.

Hypoxia

Insufficient oxygen reaching the tissues of the body.

Insight Regarding Impairment

The extent to which an individual accurately judges one's own strengths and limitations; also called metacogniton. A person's ability in this area may be judged on the basis of actions or statements regarding intended actions. Individuals with brain injury may overestimate their strengths and underestimate their limitations. For example, a person with two broken legs in casts may state that he can't walk because he's "too tired."

Intercerebral

Between the cerebral hemispheres.

Interdisciplinary Team Approach

A method of diagnosis, evaluation, and individual program planning in which two or more specialists, such as medical doctors, psychologists, recreational therapists, or social workers participate as a team with the individual and members of their family, contributing their skills, competencies, insights, and perspectives to focus on identifying the developmental needs of an individual and on devising ways to meet those needs.

Intravenous Board

A simple wooden or plastic board usually attached with tape to the forearm. It prevents bending and dislocation of the intravenous, or arterial lines.

Ipsilateral

Same side of the body.

Job Bank Service

A computerized system, developed by the Department of Labor, which maintains an up-to-date listing of job vacancies available through the State Employment Service.

Lability

Stateof having notable shifts in emotional state (e.g., uncontrolled laughing or crying).

Latency of Response/Delay

The amount of time taken to respond after the stimulus has been presented.

Learning

See Memory/Learning.

Leisure Counseling

The exploration of what types of leisure/recreation were of interest to a person before the injury and which are of interest now; how to make the best of leisure time, what recreational resources are available in the community and how to take advantage of them; and what changes have to be made to continue previous leisure pursuits.

Leisure Skills

The ability to participate in recreational activities and to independently make effective use of one's leisure time and opportunities.

Lucid Interval

A period shortly after injury when the individual was reported to have talked.

Medicaid

A joint federal/state program which provides basic health insurance for persons with disabilities, or who are poor, or receive certain governmental income support benefits (ie. Social Securiity Income or SSI) and who meet income and resource limitations. Benefits vary by state. Maybe referred to as "Title XIX" of the Social Securiity Act of 1966. Contact the state Medicaid office (listed in the blue pages of the telephone book) for more information.

Medicare

A federal health insurance program which provides acute-care coverage for people over age 65, and some individuals who receiive Social Security Disability Insurance (SSDI) benefits. Medicare has two parts: Hospital Insurance (Part A) and Medical Insurance (Part B). For more information, contact the local Social Security office (listed in the blue pages of the telephone book under "U.S. Government."

Memory

The process of organizing and storing representations of events and recalling these representations to consciousness at a later time.

Memory, Audio-Visual

Auditory memory is the ability to recall a series of numbers, lists of words, sentences, or paragraphs presented orally. Visual memory requires input of information through visuo-perceptual channels. It refers to the ability to recall text, geometric figures, maps, and photographs. A person with impaired visual memory may need frequent assistance to locate his room or home. A person with impaired auditory memory will likely require frequent reminders of orally presented task instructions.

Notably, information may be encoded in memory using words or visual images independent of the mode of presentation. Memory, Delayed The ability to recall information several minutes following presentation. There is no particular specification of the required time interval; typically it is ten minutes or more. This type of memory is most important because people are often required to recall instructions related to their medical care after hours, days, weeks, or months. For example, a person with impairments in delayed memory may forget where they have left things. Additionally, preserved information in immediate memory becomes part of delayed memory.

Memory/Learning

Change in a person's understanding or behavior due to experience or practice. Often thought of as acquisition of new information. For example, a person who learns quickly will likely remember an entire set of instructions after hearing them a single time. A person with severely-impaired learning ability will show little gain in recall after numerous repetitions. Learning and memory are interdependent. If immediate memory is poor, learning will be poor because only a portion of the information will be available for rehearsal/repetition. It is important to note that an individual may have intact learning ability, but poor delayed memory. For example, a person may learn a set of instructions after several repetitions, but forget them the next day.

Memory, Recognition

Ability to retrieve information when a stimulus cue is presented. Free recall of the information is often deficient if cues must be provided.

Memory, Remote

Information an individual correctly recalls from the past before the onset of brain injury. There is no specific requirement for the amount of elapsed time, but it is typically more than six months to a year. Preserved information from delayed memory becomes part of remote memory.

Mental Illness

A condition where there is loss of social and/or vocational skills due to impaired thought processes or emotional distress. Terms such as "mentally deranged", "crazy", "deviant" should not be used.

Metacognition

Insight into accurately judging one's own strengths and limitations, particularly with regard to cognitive skills.

Motor Control

Regulation of the timing and amount of contraction of muscles of the body to produce smooth and coordinated movement. The regulation is carried out by operation of the nervous system.

Motor Control, Fine

Delicate, intricate movements as in writing or playing a piano.

Motor Control, Gross
Large, strong movements as in chopping wood or walking.

Music Therapy
Use of music and singing to develop language and movement skills.

Neologism
Nonsense or made-up word used when speaking. The person often does not realize that the word makes no sense.

Neuro Developmental Treatment (NDT)
A therapeutic approach based on the development of movement and emphasizing the restoration of normal movement in performing functional activities.

Neurolaw
The field of jurisprudence designed to meet the challenges presented by litigation regarding injuries to the central nervous system (brain or spinal cord).

Neurologist
A physician who specializes in the nervous system and its disorders.

Neurophysiology
The study of the functions of the nervous system.

Neuropsychologist
A psychologist who specializes in evaluating (by tests) brain/behavior relationships, planning training programs to help individuals return to normal functioning and recommending alternative cognitive and behavioral strategies to minimize the effects of brain injury.

Normalization
Philosophy that developmentally disabled individuals should be exposed to patterns and conditions of daily life which are consistent with the norms of society and that training should be provided to enable persons with developmental disabilities to function appropriately in the mainstream of society.

Observational Procedure
An organized method of recording what a person does for the purpose of documenting behavior; the emphasis is usually upon productivity, behavior patterns, expressed interest, and worker interaction. Used to gain information concerning a person's overall level of functioning.

Obtunded
Mental blunting; mild to moderate reduction in alertness.

Occipital Lobe
Region in the back of the brain which processes visual information. Damage to this lobe can cause visual deficits.

Occupational Therapy (OT)
Occupational Therapy is the therapeutic of self-care, work and play activities to increase independent function, enhance development and prevent disability; may include the adaptation of a task or the environment to achieve maximum independence and to enhance the quality of life. The term

"occupation", as used in occupational therapy, refers to any activity engaged in for evaluating, specifying and treating problems interfering with functional performance.

Organization, Cognitive
Using selective attention skills, the person correctly perceives stimulus attributes or task elements, selects a strategy, monitors use of the strategy and reaches a correct solution.

Low - Level:
Able to sustain attention and appropriately switch sets. Individuals with low level organization ability usually "fall apart" in high-stress situations.

High - Level:
Able to deal with multiple piecs of information and integrate them for accomplishing relatively complex tasks. Some individuals with high level organizational abilities may still "fall apart" in high-stress situations.

Orientation, Personal
General knowledge related to oneself includes information regarding date of birth, age, name, and location of home.

Orientation, Temporal
Knowledge of the current date, day, month and year. Includes knowledge of facts related to time of day. For example, person who is disoriented who is asked to name the next meal at 4 PM might say, "breakfast."

Orthopedics
The branch of medicine devoted to the study and treatment of the skeletal system, its joints, muscles and associated structures.

Parapnasias
Use of incorrect words or word combinations.

Parenteral
Given via any type of intravenous line, including atrial line, intramuscularly, and/or subcutaneously.

Parietal Lobe
One of the two parietal lobes of the brain located behind the frontal lobe at the top of the brain.

Parietal Lobe, Right
Damage to this area can cause visuo-spatial deficits (e.g., the person may have difficulty finding their way around new or familiar places).

Parietal Lobe, Left
Damage to this area may disrupt a person's ability to understand spoken and/or written language.

Pathology
Interruption or interference of normal bodily processes or structures.

Perseveration
Refers to the inappropriate persistence of a response in a current task which may have been appropriate for a former task. Perseverations may be verbal or motoric.

Persistent Vegetative State (PVS)

A condition in which the person with no words and does not follow commands or make any response that is meaningful (persistent unawareness). The transition of a person who remains unconscious from a state of "coma" to one of "vegetative behaviors" reflects subtle changes over a period of several weeks from a condition of no response to the internal or external environment (except reflexively) to a state of wakefulness but with no indication of awareness (cortical function). A person in this state may have a range of biological responses at the subcortical level such as eye opening (with sleep and wake rhythms) and sometimes the ability to follow with their eyes. Normal levels of blood pressure and respiration (vegetative functions) are maintained automatically. The label "persistent" is not applicable until the person has been unconscious for a year or more. Also called Coma Vigil.

Personal Adjustment Training

Process of modifying behavior to conform to measurable criteria based on socially appropriate behavior; process of modifying behavior to enable one to adequately deal with one's environment.

Phonation

The production of sound by means of vocal cord vibration.

Physiatrist

Pronounced Fizz ee at' rist. A physician who specializes in physical medicine and rehabilitation. Some physiatrists are experts in neurologic rehabilitation, trained to diagnose and treat conditions which cause diisability.

Physical Therapist

The physical therapist evaluates components of movement, including: muscle strength, muscle tone, posture, coordination, endurance, and general mobility. The physical therapist also evaluates the potential for functional movement, such as ability to move in the bed, transfers and walking.

Plasticity

The ability of cellular or tissue structures and their resultant function to be influenced by an ongoing activity.

Posey Roll

A bar placed on the wheelchair to prevent a person from standing up or falling out.

Posey Vest/ Houdini Jacket

A vest worn to keep the person in bed or in the wheelchair. This is for the person's safety.

Post Traumatic Amnesia

A period of hours, weeks, days or months after the injury when a person exhibits a loss of day-to-day memory. The person is unable to store new information and therefore has a decreased ability to learn. Memory of the PTA period is never stored, therefore things that happened during that period cannot be recalled. May also be called Anterograde Amnesia.

Pre-Morbid Condition

Characteristics of an individual present before the disease or injury occurred.

Pre-Screening

The process of reviewing all available pertinent data on referrals to determine the need for additional evaluation.

Prevocational Evaluation

An assessment, prior to work training, of the individual's potential as a worker, giving special attention to one's work attitudes and habits, and evidence of personal responsibility.

Primary Care Nurse

The nurse principally responsible for the nursing care of a given individual. The primary care nurse develops and implements a care plan, participates in conferences, collaborates with the individual, the rehabilitation team, and the family, as well as evaluating the outcome of care.

Problem-Solving Skill

Ability to consider the probable factors that can influence the outcome of each of various solutions to a problem, and to select the most advantageous solution. People with deficits in this skill may become "immobilized" when faced with a problem. By being unable to think of possible solutions, they may respond by doing nothing.

Proprioception

The sensory awareness of the position of body parts with or without movement. Combination of kinesthesia and position sense.

Proximal

Next to, or nearest, the point of attachment.

Proximal Instability

Weakness of muscles of the trunk, shoulder girdle or hip girdle which causes poor posture, abnormal movement of the arms or legs and the inability to hold one's head up. Strength of muscles of the hands or legs may be normal.

Psychologist

A professional specializing in counselling, including adjustment to disability. Psychologists use tests to identify personality and cognitive functioning. This information is shared with team members to assure consistency in approaches. The psychologist may pro vide individual or group psychotherapy for the purpose of cognitive retraining, managementof behavior and the development of coping skills by the person and members of the family.

Psychometric Instruments

Standardized tests (utilizing paper and pencil) which measure mental functioning.

Psychomotor Skills

Skills that involve both mental and muscular ability such as playing sports or other activities where practice or concentration is involved.

Psychosocial Skills

Refers to the individual's adjustment to the injury (and resulting disability) and one's ability to relate to others. Includes feelings about self, sexuality and the resulting behaviors.

P.A.

Physician's Assistant.

P.T.

Physical Therapist

PTA

See post traumatic amnesia.

Quadriparesis

Weakness of all four limbs.

Quadriplegia

Paralysis of all four limbs (from the neck down). British authors often use the prefix "tetra" to mean four, so they may describe a person as having tetraplegia.

Quality of Life

A rating of what kind of existence a person experiences. In estimating the quality of life the following items are usually considered: 1) mobility and activities of daily life; 2) living arrangements; 3) social relationships; 4) work and leisure activities; 5) present satisfaction; and 6) future prospects.

R.T.

Respiratory Therapist.

Reasoning, Abstract

Requires that the individual recognize a phrase that has multiple meanings and select the meaning most appropriate to a given situation. The term "abstract" typically refers to concepts not readily apparent from the physical attributes of an object or situation.

Reasoning, Association

A skill dependent on a person's ability to determine the relationship between objects and concepts. A person may touch a hot stove, failing to realize that pain is associated with touching a heated burner. Similarly, given a knife, spoon, fork, and baseball, a person may not be able to discriminate which of the objects "does not belong."

Reasoning, Categorization

The ability to sort or group objects and concepts based on the shared attribute(s) and apply a label depicting the attribute(s). Task difficulty is greater in circumstances requiring formulation of new categories. People may have difficulty sorting clothes or choosing items for a balanced meal. Categorization is similar to association in that the relationship between objects or concepts must be understood. However, categorization requires an extra step; the ability to provide a label describing the group of objects or concepts.

Reasoning, Organization

The ability to arrange or group information in a manner which improves task efficiency. People who lack organizational skills often demonstrate a sense of purposelessness and have difficulty effectively utilizing non-structured time. They have difficulty completing a puzzle or arranging materials to cook or shower.

Recreation Therapist

Individual within the facility responsible for developing a program to assist persons with disabilities plan and manage their leisure activities; may also schedule specific activities and coordinate the program with existing community resources.

Registry

A clinical or service oriented system used to: 1) identify individuals who are eligible for services, 2) evaluate treatment methods, and 3) monitor outcomes.

Rehabilitation Counselor

Also called Vocational Counselor. A specialist in social and vocational issues who helps the person with a disability develop the skills and aptitudes necessary for return to productive activity and the community.

Rehabilitation Facility

Agency of multiple, coordinated services designed to minimize for the individual the disabling effects of one's physical, mental, social, and/or vocational difficulties and to help realize individual potential.

Rehabilitation Objective

A goal of the comprehensive restoration of an individual to the best possible level of functioning following a physical, mental, or emotional disorder.

Rehabilitation Process

A planned, orderly sequence of services related to the total needs of the person with a disability and designed to assist one to realize maximum potential for useful and productive activity.

Remediation

The process of decreasing a disability by challenging the individual to improve deficient skills.

Respite Care

A means for taking over the care of a person temporarily (a few hours up to a few days) to provide a period of relief for the primary caregiver.

Response Control

Development of the ability to recognize and suppress abnormal behaviors in one's self. Two behaviors fall within this category: impulse control, and perseveration.

Respiratory Therapist

The respiratory therapist is concerned with helping the person breathe adequately by use of various machines as well as techniques to keep the airway clear of secretions.

Retrograde Amnesia

Inability to recall events prior to the accident; may be a specific span of time or type of information.

S.T.

See Speech and Hearing Therapist.

Scotoma

Area of blindness of varying size anywhere within the visual fields.

Seizure

An uncontrolled discharge of nerve cells which may spread to other cells nearby or throughout the entire brain. It usually lasts only a few minutes. It may be associated with loss of consciousness, loss of bowel and bladder control and tremors. May also cause aggressive or other behavioral change.

Sensorimotor

Refers to all aspects of movement and sensation and the interaction of the two.

Shunt

A procedure to draw off excessive fluid in the brain. A surgically-placed tube running from the ventricles which deposits fluid into either the abdominal cavity, heart or large veins of the neck.

Single Trait Work Samples

Assesses a single worker trait or characteristic. It may have relevance to a specific job or many jobs, but it is intended to assess a single, isolated factor.

Skill Remediation

A process in which the aim is to improve skills that have been imperfectly or inadequately learned.

Social Adjustment Group

A structured group experience that offers individuals opportunities for the redirection of energies toward positive social goals, raising of levels of aspiration, and/or reduction of maladaptive behavior patterns.

Social Adjustment Training

Structured program designed to assist the disabled individual to interact with individuals and groups within the community in an acceptable manner.

Social Assessment

A social assessment includes general background data, description of family or other support group resources — including emotional, financial and environment resources, their availability to the person, and the person's position and role in the family (child, parent, spouse) — and educational and employment history. Also included are such topics as interests, life-style, friendships, goals, ambitions, personality traits, positive and/or negative relationships and previous problems (such as medical, psychiatric, drug abuse, alcohol). The assessment attempts to reveal the individuals's and the family's level of under standing of the person's current condition, probable long-range outcome, expectations of rehabilitation, degree of disruption in family functioning that the disability has produced, and the ability and interest of the individual and family members to adjust to changed circum stances.

Social Worker

The social worker serves as a liaison between the professional team and other parties concerned with the person, including: the family, funding sources, friends and representatives of past or future placements. An important role of the social worker is to help ensure that if home placement does not materialize, or if home placement is not indicated, the social worker provides assistance to the person and family for finding other alternatives.

Somatic

Relating to, or affecting the body.

Somatosensory

Sensory activity having its origin elsewhere than in the special sense organs (such as eyes and ears) and conveying information to the brain about the state of the body proper and its immediate environment.

Spasticity

An involuntary increase in muscle tone (tension) that occurs following injury to the brain or spinal cord, causing the muscles to resist being moved. Charac teristics may include increase in deep tendon reflexes, resistance to passive stretch, clasp knife phenomenon, and clonus.

Special

Describes that which is different or uncommon about any person. This term should not be used to describe persons with disabilities (except when citing laws or regulations).

Specialty Services

Categories identified by the National Head Injury Foundation (NHIF) to classify frequently requested services. These services include: respirator-dependent, substance abuse, driver education, evaluation, visually-impaired and Spanish translation.

Specific Learning Disability

Permanent condition that affects the way individuals with average or above-average intelligence take in, retain, and express information. The term "specific" is preferred, because it emphasizes that only certain learning processes are affected.

Speech and Hearing Therapist

The speech pathologist and audiologist identifies problem areas of visual (seeing) and auditory (hearing) comprehension, attention, memory (recent and past), language skills, writing skills and reading skills. The information gathered by the speech and hearing specialist is valuable to other team members; for example, whether or not to use reading as a means of communicating information to the individual. The speech therapist provides instruction and practice in improving skills in comprehension and communication.

Speech-Language Pathology Services

A continuum of services including prevention, identification, diagnosis, consultation, and treatment regarding speech, language, oral and pharyngeal sensorimotor function.

Spontaneous Recovery

The recovery which occurs as damage to body tissues heals. This type of recovery occurs with or without rehabilitation and it is very difficult to know how much improvement is spontaneous and how much is due to rehabilitative interventions. However, when the recovery is guided by an experienced rehabilitation team, complications can be anticipated and minimized; the return of function can be channeled in useful directions and in progressive steps so that the eventual outcome is the best that is possible.

Supervision, Close

Refers to the assistance provided when an individual requires no physical help but requires another person nearby for safety. Assistant stands close to person, ready to give assistance if needed.

Supervision, Distant

Assistant can see the person and offer verbal assistance but is not close enough to touch the person.

Support Group

A group established for families and/or persons with disabilities to discuss the problems they may be having in coping with their life situation and to seek solutions to these problems.

Supported Employment

Competitive work in integrated work settings for individuals with severe disabilities for whom competitive employment has not traditionally occurred, or for whom competitive employment has been interrupted as a result of severe disability, and who, because of the disability, need ongoing support services to perform that work.

Surveillance System

A means of gathering data; generally has publich health emphasis containing only descriptive information used to assess the magnitude of particular types of health problems, and is geared toward prevention of the problem.

Synergy (movement)

Combined action of two or more muscles to form a pattern of movement.

Tactile Defensiveness

Being overly sensitive to touch;withdrawing, crying, yelling or striking when one is touched.

Tactile Discrimination

The ability to differentiate information received through the sense of touch. Sharp/dull discrimination - ability to distinguish between sharp and dull stimuli; Two-point discrimination - the ability to recognize two points applied to the skin simultaneously as distinct from one single point.

Team, Inter-disciplinary

A type of team functioning in which the persons representing each discipline (field of study) have a voice in establishing priorities for the goals to be undertaken by members of the team.

Team, Multi-disciplinary

A type of team functioning in which the persons representing each discipline (field of study) set their own goals for evaluating and treating the person and inform other team members of the results as they occur.

Team, Trans-disciplinary

A type of team functioning in which the persons representing each discipline (field of study) are encouraged to deal with problems or issues as they occur during daily interactions with the person even though the intervention used may fall within the primary domain of another discipline.

TEDS

See Support Hose

Telegraphic Speech

Speech which sounds like a telegram. Only the main words of a sentence (nouns, verbs) are present; the small words (ifs, ands, buts,) are missing. This type of speech often gets the message across.

Temporal Lobes

There are two temporal lobes, one on each side of the brain located at about the level of the ears. These lobes allow a person to tell one smell from another and one sound from another. They also help in sorting new information and are believed to be responsible for short-term memory.

Right Lobe

Mainly involved in visual memory (i.e., memory for pictures and faces).

Left Lobe

Mainly involved in verbal memory (i.e., memory for words and names).

Time Study

Detailed, scientific analysis of time taken by a worker to perform each segment of a specific task/job, and the hand and body movements made in performing the task/job. Such a study may be made for the purpose of determining the most efficient method for doing the task/job, or to evaluate the task/job to establish a work standard or to set a wage.

Tracheostomy

A temporary surgical opening at the front of the throat providing access to the trachea or windpipe to assist in breathing.

Tracking, Visual

Visually following an object as it moves through space.

Training Environment

Refers to the setting in which the emphasis is on the learning and acquisition of skills or competencies.

Transfer

Moving one's body between wheelchair and bed, toilet, mat, or car with or without the assistance of another person.

Treatment Modalities

Various therapy techniques.

Treatment Protocol

The written treatment plan specifying the procedures to be followed by the treatment team.

Tremor, Intention

Course, rhythmical movements of a body part that become intensified the harder one tries to control them.

Tremor, Resting

Rhythmical movements present at rest and may be diminished during voluntary movement.

Unilateral

Pertaining to only one side.

Unilateral Neglect

Paying little or no attention to things on one side of the body. This usually occurs on the side opposite from the location of the injury to the brain because nerve fibers from the brain typically cross before innervating body stru ctures. In extreme cases, the person may not bathe, dress or acknowledge one side of the body.

Vegetative State

Return of wakefulness but not accompanied by cognitive function; eyes open to verbal stimuli; does not localize motor responses; autonomic functions preserved. Sleep-wake cycles exist. See Persistent Vegetative State.

Ventricles, Brain

Four natural cavities in the brain which are filled with cerebrospinal fluid. The outline of one or more of these cavities may change when a space-occupying lesion (hemorrhage, tumor) has developed in a lobe of the brain.

Verbal Ability

Composed of verbal understanding and verbal fluency. Verbal understanding is the ability of an individual to understand the subtleties and meaning of words; verbal fluency is the ability to imagine, process and say words without associating them with any particular object. Also the ability to communicate by talking, writing, listening and reading.

Verbal Apraxia

Impaired control of proper sequencing of muscles used in speech (tongue, lips, jaw muscles, vocal cords). These muscles are not weak but their control is defective. Speech is labored and characterized by sound reversals, additions and word approximations.

Verbal Fluency

The ability to produce words.

Visual Field Defect

Inability to see objects located in a specific region of the field of view ordinarily received by each eye. Often the blind region includes everything in the right half or left half of the visual field.

Vocational Counseling

Process of assisting a person to under stand vocational liabilities and assets, provide occupational information to assist one in choosing an occupation suitable to one's interests and liabilities.

Vocational Education

Courses of study, under supervision and control, which lead to proficiency in specific trades or business occupations.

Vocational Evaluation

A comprehensive process that systematically utilizes work, real or simulated, as the focal point for assessment and vocational exploration, the purpose of which is to assist individuals in vocational development. Vocational evaluation incorporates medical, psychological, social, vocational, educational, cultural, and economic data in the at tainment of the goals of the evaluation process.

Vocational Rehabilitation Process

Providing, in a coordinated manner, those services deemed appropriate to the needs of a person with a disability, and designed to achieve objectives directed toward the realization of the individual's maximum physical, social, mental, and vocational potential.

Wagner-O'Day

Common name for Public Law 92-28 which directs the purchase by the Federal Government of selected commodities and services from qualified workshops serving blind and other severely disabled individuals, with the objective of increasing the employment opportunities for these individuals.

Work Activity Center

A workshop, or physically-separate department of a workshop, having a planned, identifiable program designed exclusively to provide therapeutic activity for workers whose physical or mental impairment is so severe as to make their production inconsequential.

Work Adjustment

An individualized, structured and planned, closely supervised, remedial work experience designed to promote the acquisition of good work habits, to increase physical and emotional tolerance for work activity and interpersonal relationships, and to modify aptitudes and behaviors which inhibit the satisfactory performance of work.

Worker's Compensation

See Terms and Definitions Related to Insurance.

Worker Functions

The functioning of the worker in relationship to a specific set of tasks. A combination of the highest function which the worker performs in relation to data, people, and things, expresses the total level of complexity of the job/worker situation.

Workmen's Compensation

Insurance programs, under state auspices or control, except for Federal employees and certain maritime workers, to provide financial resources for medical care and lost wages and earning power resulting from industrial accidents, and from illnesses resulting from employment.

Work Sample

A well defined work activity involving tasks, materials, and tools which are identical or similar to those in an actual job or cluster of jobs. It is used to assess an individual's vocational aptitude, worker characteristics, and vocational interest.

61– Glossary 92

Americans with Disability Act (ADA) Terms

ABA

The Architectural Barriers Act of 1968. P.L. 90-480, as amended.

Affirmative Action

This concept involves a commitment to positive action to accomplish the purposes of a program. It may involve goals or timetables and specifically outlined steps that will be pursued to assure that objectives are attained. The ADA does not mandate affirmative action for disabled people. Rather, the ADA requires that covered entities ensure "non-discrimination". In the context of civil rights for disabled people, affirmative action must be taken under Section 503 of the Rehabilitation Act, which requires affirmative steps and positive outreach by federal contractors in employment considerations.

Auxillary Aids

Devices or services that compensate for a disabling condition. The term includes qualified interpreters or other means of communications (such as telecommunica tions devices for the deaf — TDDs) for hearing- impaired people; qualified readers, taped texts or other devices for sight-impaired people; adaptive equipment; and other similar services and actions.

Equal Employment Opportunity Commission

The U.S. Equal Employment Opportunity Commission (EEOC) enforces the non-discrimination requirements in Title I (employment) of the ADA.

Equal Opportunity

The elimination of unfair and unnecessary discrimination. Equal opportunity for qualified disabled people is an objective of the ADA. This goal translates into the achievement of accessi bility, the provision of benefits, services and aids that are equally effective for disabled and non-disabled people, and programs and activities that are otherwise free from discrimination based on disability.

Individual With A Disability

This term refers to any person who: (1) has a physical or mental impairment that substantially limits one or more major life activities (i.e., caring for one's self, performing manual tasks, walking, seeing, hearing, speaking, breathing, learning and working); (2) has a record of such an impairment (has a history of, or has been misclassified that substantially limits one or more major life activities); or (3) is regarded as having such an impairment.

Minimum Guidelines & Requirements Accessible Design (MGRAD)

Issued by the Architectural and Transportation Barriers Compliance Board, which are the basis for federal accessibility standards. Buildings, facilities and vehicles are considered to be in compliance with the ADA if they follow the architectural, design and communications standards contained in the MGARAD.

Non-discrimination

Non-discrimination is mandated by the ADA. No otherwise qualified disabled individual can, solely by reason of his or her disability, be subjected to discrimination. Covered entities are required under the ADA to ensure non-dis crimination by providing accessibility, equal opportunity and full partici-pation in employment and public facilities and services.

Qualified Individual with a Disability

With respect to employment, a disabled person who, with or without reasonable accommodation, can perform the essential functions of the job in question; and (2) with respect to public services, an individual who, with or without reasonable modifications to rules, policies or practices, the removal of architectural, communication or transportation barriers, or the provision of auxiliary aids and services, meets the essential eligibility requirements for the receipt of services or participation in the program or activity.

Rehabilitation Act of 1973

Prohibits federal agencies and their grantees and contractors from discriminating against people based on disability in employment, programs and activities. Title V of the rehabilitation Act, 29 U.S.C. 791 et. seq., is the legislative forerunner of the ADA indeveloping concepts of "qualified individual with a disability" and "reasonable accommodation".

Terms and Definitions Related to Insurance

Accident

An event causing loss, which takes place without being expected. In most cases the accident can be characterized with regard to time and place of occurrence.

Blanket Medical Expense

A provision which entitles the insured person to collect up to a maximum established in the policy for all hospital and medical expenses incurred, without any limitation on individual types of medical expenses.

Coinsurance

A policy provision frequently found in major medical insurance, by which both the insured person and the insurer share the covered losses under a policy in a specified ratio.

Comprehensive Major Medical Insurance

A policy designed to give the protection offered by both a basic and a major medical health insurance policy. It is characterized by a low deductible amount, a coinsurance feature, and high maximum benefits.

Contributory

A group insurance plan issued to an employer under which both the employer and employee contribute to the cost of the plan; 75% of the eligible employees must be insured.

Double Indemnity

A policy provision usually associated with death, which doubles payment of a designated benefit when certain kinds of accidents occur.

Morbidity

The incidence and severity of sicknesses and accidents in a well-defined class or classes of people.

Nondisabling Injury

An injury which may require medical care, but does not result in loss of working time or income.

Partial Disability

The result of an illness or injury which prevents an insured from performing one or more of the functions of his/her regular job.

Rider

A document which amends the policy or certificate. It may increase or decrease benefits, waive the conditions of coverage, or in any other way amend the original contract.

Total Disability

An illness or injury that prevents an insured person from continuously performing every duty pertaining to his/her occupation or engaging in any other type of work.

Brain Injury Association
State Network Listing

**The following states have become fully chartered associations
under the Brain Injury Association:**

ALABAMA Head Injury Foundation
P.O. Box 550008
Birmingham, AL 35255

Phone: (205) 328-3505
(800) 433-8002 (in state)

ARIZONA Head Injury Foundation
630 N. Craycroft Road, Suite 139
Tucson, AZ 85711-1441

Phone: (602) 747-7140
(800) 432-3465 (in state)

ARKANSAS Head Injury Foundation
106 Kansas
Little Rock, AR 72118

Phone: (501) 771-5011
(800) 235-2443

CALIFORNIA Head Injury Foundation
P.O. Box 160786
Sacramento, CA 95816-0786

Phone: (916) 442-1710
(800) 457-CHIF

COLORADO Head Injury Foundation
5601 S. Broadway, Suite 350
Littleton, CO 80121

Phone: (303) 730-7112
(800) 955-2443 (in state)

CONNECTICUT Traumatic Brain Injury Association
1800 Silas Deane Highway, Suite 224
Rocky Hill, CT 06067

Phone: (203) 721-8111
(800) 278-8242 (in state)

DELAWARE Head Injury Foundation
P.O. Box 9876
Newark, DE 19714

Phone: (302) 475-2286

FLORIDA Head Injury Association
North Broward Medical Center
201 E. Sample Road
Pompano Beach, FL 33064

Phone: (305) 786-2400
(800) 992-3442 (in state)

Brain Injury Association of GEORGIA
1447 Peachtree Street NE, Suite 810
Atlanta, GA 30309

Phone (404) 817-7577
Fax (404) 817-7521

BIA / ILLINOIS
1127 S. Mannheim Road, Suite 213
Westchester, IL 60154

Phone: (708) 344-4646
(800) 699-6443 (in state)

Head Injury Foundation / INDIANA
5506 East 16th Street, Suite B5   Phone: (317) 356-7722
Indianapolis, IN 46218-4930   (800) 407-4246 Helpline

Brain Injury Association of IOWA
2101 Kimball Avenue, LL7   Phone: (319) 291-3552
Waterloo, IA 50702   (800) 475-4442 (in state)

Head Injury Association of KANSAS & Greater Kansas City
1100 Pennsylvania, Suite 305   Phone: (816) 842-8607
Kansas City, MO 64105-1336   (800) 783-1356

Brain Injury Association of KENTUCKY
3910 Dupont Square South, Suite D   Phone:(502) 899-7141
Louisville, KY 40207-4648   (800) 592-1117

LOUISIANA Head Injury Foundation
217 Buffwood Drive   Phone (504) 775-2780
Buker, LA 70714-3755

MAINE Head Injury Foundation
424 Western Avenue   Phone: (207) 626-0022
Augusta, ME 04330   (800) 275-1233

Brain Injury Association of MARYLAND
916 S. Rolling Road   Phone: (410) 747-7758
Baltimore, MD 21228   (800) 221-NHIF (in state)

MASSACHUSETTS Head Injury Association
Denholm Building   Phone: (508) 795-0244
484 Main Street, #325   (800) 242-0030 (in state)
Worcester, MA 01608

MICHIGAN Head Injury Alliance
8137 W. Grand River, Suite A   Phone: (810) 229-5880
Brighton, MI 48116   (800) 772-4323 (in state)

Brain Injury Association of MINNESOTA
12 Colonial Office Park   Phone: (612) 644-1121
2700 University Avenue West   (800) 669-MHIA (in state)
St. Paul, MN 55114

MISSISSIPPI Head Injury Association
P.O. Box 55912   Phone: (601) 981-1021
Jackson, MS 39296-5912   (800) 641-6442

MISSOURI Head Injury Association
P.O. Box 37070   Phone: (417) 888-7708
St. Louis, MO 63141   (800) 377-6442 (in state)

Brain Injury Association of MONTANA
Inst. for Health & Human Services
Eastern Montana College, Room 235
1500 N. 30th Street
Billings, MT 59101-0298

Phone: (406) 657-2077
(800) 241-6442 (in state)

NEBRASKA Head Injury Association
P.O. Box 397
Route 1, Box 132
Milford, NE 68405

Phone: (402) 761-2781
(800) 743-4781 (in state)

NHIF/NEW HAMPSHIRE Association
2 1/2 Beacon Street, Suite 171
Concord, NH 03301

Phone:(603) 225-8400

NEW JERSEY Head Injury Association
1090 King George Post Road #708
Edison, NJ 08837-3722

Phone: (908) 738-1002
(800) 669-4323 (in state)

NEW MEXICO Head Injury Foundation
2819 Richmond, N.E.
Albuquerque, NM 87107

Phone: (505) 889-8008
(800) 279-7480 (in state)

NEW YORK State Head Injury Association
10 Colvin Avenue
Albany, NY 12206

Phone: (518) 459-7911
(800) 228-8201 (in state)

Brain Injury Association of NORTH CAROLINA
133 Fayetteville Street Mall, Suite 310
Raleigh, NC 27601

Phone (919) 833-9634
(800) 377-1464 (in state)

Head Injury Association of NORTH DAKOTA
2111 E. Main Avenue, Suite 14
West Fargo, ND 58708

Phone: (701) 281-0527
(800) 279-6344 (in state)

The OHIO Head Injury Association
1335 Dublin Road, Suite 50A
Columbus, OH 43215-1000

Phone: (614) 481-7100
(800) 686-9563 (in state)

Brain Injury Association of OKLAHOMA
P.O. Box 88
Hillsdale, OK 73743-0088

Phone: (405) 635-2237
(800) 765-6809 (in state)

OREGON Head Injury Foundation
1118 Lancaster Drive NE, Ste 345
Salem, OR 97301

Phone: (503) 585-0855
(800) 544-5243 (in state)

SOUTH CAROLINA Head Injury Association
P.O. Box 1945
Orangeburg, SC 29116

Phone: (803) 533-1613
(800) 767-9701 (in state)

Brain Injury Association of TENNESSEE
699 W. Main Street, Ste 208   Phone: (615) 264-3052
Hendersonville, TN 37075   (800) 480-6693

TEXAS Head Injury Association
Plaza 290 Office Building, Suite 301   Phone: (512) 467-6872
6633 East Highway 290   (800) 392-0040 (in state)
Austin, TX 78723

UTAH Head Injury Association
1800 S. West Temple, Suite 203, Box 22   Phone: (801) 484-2240
Salt Lake City, UT 84115   (800) 281-8442 (in state)

VERMONT Association/NHIF
P.O. Box 1837, Station A   Phone: (802) 446-3017
Rutland, VT 05773

VIRGINIA Head Injury Foundation
3212 Cutshaw Avenue, Suite 315   Phone: (804) 355-5748
Richmond, VA 23230   (800) 334-8443 (in state)

Brain Injury Association of WASHINGTON
300 120th Avenue, N.E.   Phone: (206) 451-0000
Building 3, Room 131   (800) 523-LIFT (in state)
Bellevue, WA 98005

WEST VIRGINIA Head Injury Foundation
P.O. Box 574   Phone: (304) 766-4892
Institute, WV 25112-0574   (800) 356-6443 (in state)

WISCONSIN Brain Trauma Association
735 N. Water Street, Suite 701   Phone: (414) 271-7463
Milwaukee, WI 53202   (800) 882-9282 (in state)

WYOMING Brain Injury Association
246 South Center, Suite 206   Phone: (307) 473-1767
Casper, WY 82601   (800) 643-6457 Nationwide

Child/Adolescent Brain Injury References

Books

Begali, V. (1992). Head injury in children and adolescents (2nd ed.). Brandon, VT: CPPC.

Berrol, S., & Rosenthal, M. (Eds.). (1991). The Journal of Head Trauma Rehabilitation: School Reentry Following Head Injury, 6(1).

Blosser, J.L. & DePompei, R. (1994). Pediatric traumatic brain injury: Proactive intervetion. San Diego, CA: Singular Publishing Group.

Gerring, J. & Carney, J. (1992). Head trauma; strategies for educational reintegration, 2nd edition. San Diego, CA Singular Publishing Group.

Lehr, E. (Ed.). (1990). Psychological management of head injuries in children and adolescents. Rockville, MD: Aspen.

Rosen, C. D., & Gerring, J. P. (1986). Head trauma: Educational reintegration. Boston: College-Hill Press.

Rosenthal, M., Griffith, E., Bond, M., & Miller, J.D. (Eds.) (1990), Rehabilitation of the adult and child with traumatic brain Injury. Philadelphia: F.A. Davis.

Savage, R. and Wolcott, G. (1994). Educational dimensions of acquired brain injury. Austin, TX: Pro-Ed.

Shapiro, K. (Ed.) Pediatric head trauma. New York: Futura.

Walsh, K. (1987). Neuropsychology A Clinical Approach. Edinburgh: Churchill Livingstone.

Wiederholt, J.L. (Ed.). (1987). Journal of Learning Disabilities, 20(8, 9 & 10).

Williams, J.M., & Kay, T. (1991). Head Injury: A Family Matter, Grand Rapids: P.H.Brooks.

Ylvisaker, M. (Ed.). (1985). Head injury rehabilitation: Children and adolescents. San Diego:College-Hill Press.

Manuals

Lash, M. (1992). When Your Child Goes to School After an Injury. Boston, MA: Exceptional Parent.

Lash, M. (1990). When Your Child is Seriously Injured..the Emotional Impact on Families. Boston, MA: Exceptional Parent.

Mira, M., Tyler, J., & Trucker, B. (1988). Traumatic head injury in children: A guide for schools. Kansas City, KS: University of Kansas Medical Center, Children's Rehabilitation Unit.

Tyler, J. (1990). Traumatic head injury in school-aged children: A training manual for educational personnel. Kansas City, KS: University of Kansas Medical Center, Children's Rehabilitation Unit.

Videotapes

"Returning to School Following Traumatic Brain Injury" Research and Training Center, Medical College of Richmond, VA. Telephone (804) 786-7290

"Perspectives on Traumatic Brain Injury" Dept. of Special Education, University of Kansas, Lawrence, KS. Telephone (913) 588-5943.

"School Re-entry for the Student with Traumatic Brain Injury" University Hospital School, Iowa City, Iowa. ATTN: Sue Pearson. Telephone (319) 356-1172

"Families Living with Brain Injury" University Hospital School, Iowa City, Iowa. ATTN: Sue Pearson. Telephone (319) 356-1172.

Articles

Cognitive/Academic

Boll, T. J. (1983). Minor head injury in children - out of sight but not out of mind. Journal of Clinical Psychology, 12, 74-80.

Chadwick, O., Rutter, M., Thompson, J., & Shaffer, D. (1981). Intellectual performance and reading ability after localized head injury in childhood. Journal of Child Psychology and Psychiatry, 22, 117-39.

Goldstein, F. C. & Levin, H. C. (1985). Intellectual and academic outcome following closed head injury in children and adolescents: Research strategies and empirical findings. Developmental Neuropsychology, 1, (3), 195-214.

Levin, H. S.., Eisenberg, H. M., Wigg, N. R., & Kobayashi, K. (1982). Memory and intellectual ability after head injury in children and adolescents. Neurosurgery, 11, 668-73.

Shaffer, D., Bijur, P., Chadwick, O., & Rutter, M. (1980). Head injury and later reading disability. Journal of the American Academy of Child Psychiatry, !9, 592-610.

Telzrow, C. (1987). Management of academic and educational problems in head injury. Journal of Learning Disabilities, 20 (9), 536-45.

Wood, R. L. (1988). Attention disorders in brain injury rehabilitation. Journal of Learning Disabilities, 21 (6), 327-32.

Ylvisaker, M. (1989). Cognitive and psychosocial outcome following head injury. In Hoff, J.T., Anderson, T.E., & Cole, T.M. (Eds.)., Mild to Moderate Head Injury. London: Blackwell Scientific.

Behavioral

Deaton, A. V. (1987). Behavior change strategies for children and adolescents with severe brain injury. Journal of Learning Disabilities, 20 (10), 581-89.

Filley, C. M., Cranberg, M.D., Alexander, M. P., & Hart, E. J. (1987). Neurobehavioral outcome after closed head injury in childhood and adolescence. Archives of Neurology, 44, 194-98.

Fletcher, J.M., Ewing-Cobbs, L., Miner, M.E., Levin, H.S. & Eisenberg, H.M. (1990). Behavioral Change After Closed Head Injury in Children. Journal of Consulting and Clinical Psychology, 58, 93-98.

Rutter, M., Chadwick, O., & Shaffer, D. (1983). Head injury. In Rutter, M. (Ed.), Developmental Neuropsychiatry. New York: Guilford.

Physical Recovery

Brink, J. D., Imbus, C., & Woo-Sam, J. (1980). Physical recovery after severe closed head trauma in children and adolescents. Journal of Pediatrics, 97, 721-727.

Family

DePompei, R. & Blosser, J. Families of Children with Traumatic Brain Injury as Advocates in School Reentry. Neurorehabilitation, 1(2), 29-37.

Martin, D. A. (1988). Children and adolescents with TBI: Impact on the family. Journal of Learning Disabilities, 21 (8), 464-70.

School Re-entry

Blosser, J. & DePompei, R. (1989). The head injured student returns to school: Recognizing and treating deficits. Topics in Language Disorders, 9 (2), 67-77.

Burns, P.G. & Gianutsos, R. (1987). Re-entry of the head-injured survivor into the educational system: First steps. Journal of Community Health Nursing, 4, 145-52.

Jacobs, M.P. (1989). Head injured students in the public schools: A model program. The Forum, 14 (4), 9-11.

Lash, M., & Scarpino, C. (1993). School reintegration for children with traumatic brain injuries: conflicts between medical and educational systems. Neurorehabilitation, 3(3), 13-25.

Lehr, E. & Savage, R. (1992). Community and school integration from a developmental perspective. in Keutzer, J, (Ed.), Community Integration Baltimore: Paul Brooks.

Mira, M. P. & Tyler, J. S. (1991). Students with traumatic brain injury: Making the transition from hospital to school. Focus on Exceptional Children, 23 (5), 1-12.

Reynolds, C.R. (1986). Transactional models of intellectual development, yes, deficit models of process remediation, no. School Psychology Review, 15 (2), 256-260.

Savage, R. C. & Carter, R. (1984, Nov/Dec). Re-entry: The head injured student returns to school. Cognitive Rehabilitation, 28-33.

Tucker, B.F. & Colson, S.E. (1992). Traumatic brain injury: An overview of school re-entry. Intervention in School and Clinic, 27 (4), 198-206.

Ylvisaker, M., Hartwick, P., & Stevens, M. (1991). School re-entry following head injury: Managing transition from hospital to school. Journal of Head Trauma Rehabilitation, 6 (1), 10-22.

Assessment

Bernstein, J.H., & Waber, D.P. (1990). Developmental neuropsychological assessment: the systematic approach. In Boulton, A.A., Baker, G.B., & Hiscock, M. (Eds.), Neuromethods: Vol. 17, Neuropsychology. Clifton, NJ: Humana Press.

Telzrow, C. F. (1989). Neuropsychological applications of common educational and psychological tests. In Reynolds, C.R., & Fletcher-Janzen, E., (Eds.) Handbook of Clinical Child Neuropsychology. New York, NY: Plenum.

Legal Aspects

Martin, R. (1988). Legal challenges in educating traumatic brain injured students. Journal of Learning Disabilities, 21 (8), 471-75.

Savage, R.C. (1991). Identification, classification, and placement of traumatically brain injured students. Journal of Head Trauma. Rehabilitation, 6 (1), 1-9.

Professional Issues

Haak, R.A. (1989). Establishing neuropsychology in a school setting: organization, problems, and benefits. In Reynolds, C.R., & Fletcher-Janzen, E., (Eds.), Handbook of Clinical Child Neuropsychology, New York, N.Y: Plenum.

Hynd, G.W., Quackenbush, R., & Obrzut, J.E. (1980). Training School Psychologists in Neuropsychology: Current Practices and Trends. Journal of School Psychology, 18, 148-153.

Leavell, C., & Lewandowski, L. (1988). Neuropsychology in the schools: a survey report. School Psychology Review, 17, 147-155.

McMahon, B.T. (1991). Ethics in business practices. In McMahon, B.T. & Shaw, L.R. (Eds.), Work Worth Doing: Advances in Brain Injury Rehabilitation. Orlando Fl.: Paul Deutsch.

Mira, M.P., Meck, N.E., & Tyler, J.S. (1988). School psychologists' knowledge of traumatic brain injury: Implications for training. Diagnostique, 13(2-4), 174-180.

Incidence and Service Delivery

Gans, B.M. & DiScala, C. (1991). Rehabilitation of severely injured children. Western Journal of Medicine, 154, 566-568.

Lescohier, I., & DiScala, C. (1993). Blunt trauma in children: causes and outcomes of head versus extracranial injury. Pediatrics, 91 (4), 721-725.

Osberg, J.S., DiScala, C., Gans, B.M. (1990). Utilization of inpatient rehabilitation services among traumatically injured children discharged from pediatric trauma centers. American Journal of Physical Medicine and Rehabilitation, 69, (2), 67-72.

References and Resources

Brown, G., Chadwick, O., Shaffer, D., Rutter, M., & Traub, M. (1981). A prospective study of children with head injuries. III. Psychiatric sequelae. Psychological Medicine, 11, 63-78.

Campbell T.F., & Dollaghan, C.A. (1990). Expressive language recovery in severely brain injured children and adolescents. Journal of Speech and Hearing Disorders. 55(3), 567-581.

Chapman, S., Culhane, K., Levin, H., Harward, H., Mendelsohn, D., Ewing-Cobbs, L., Fletcher, J., & Bruce, D. (1992). Narrative discourse after closed head injury in children and adolescents. Brain and Language, 43, 42-65.

Cooper, J.A., & Flowers, C.R. (1987). Children with a history of acquired aphasia: Residual language and academic impairments. Journal of Speech and Hearing Disorders, 52, 251-262.

Dennis, M. (1992). Word-finding in children and adolescents with a history of brain injury. Topics in Language Disorders. 13, 66-82.

Dennis, M., & Barnes, M. (1990). Knowing the meaning, getting the point, bridging the gap, and carrying the message: Aspects of discourse following closed head injury in childhood and adolescence. Brain and Language, 39, 428-446.

Dennis, M., & Lovett, M. (1990). Discourse ability in children after brain damage. In Y. Joanette & H.H. Brownell (Eds.), Discourse ability and brain damage: Theoretical and empirical perspectives (pp. 199-223). New York: Springer Verlag

Ewing-Cobbs, L., Levin, H.S., Eisenberg, H.M., & Fletcher, J.M. (1987). Language functions following closed head injury in children and adolescents. Journal of Clinical and Experimental Neuropsychology, 9, 575-592.

Ewing-Cobbs, L., Miner, M., Fletcher, J.M., & Levin, H.S. (1989). Intellectual, motor, and language squelae following closed head injury in infants and preschoolers. Journal of Pediatric Psychology, 14(4), 513-544

Fletcher, J.M., Ewing-Cobbs, L., Miner, M., & Levin, H.S. (1990). Behavioral changes after closed head injury in children. Journal of Consulting and Clinical Psychology, 58, 93-98.

Jordan, F.M., Ozanne, A.E., & Murdoch, B.E. (1988). Long-term speech and language disorders subsequent to closed head injury in children. Brain Injury, 2, 179-185.

Jordan, F.M., Murdoch, B.E., & Buttsworth, D.L. (1991). Closed-head-injured children's performance on narrative tasks. Journal of Speech and Hearing Research, 34, 572-582.

Perrott, S.B., Taylor, H.G., & Montes, J.L. (1991). Neuropsychological sequelae, familial stress, and environmental adaptation following pediatric head injury. Developmental Neuropsychology, 7, 69-86.

Patterson, L. (1988). Sensitivity to emotional cues and social behavior in children and adolescents after head injury. Ph.D. Dissertation, University of Minnesota.

Rutter, M., Chadwick, O., & Shaffer, D. (1983). Head injury. In M. Ruttet (Ed.), Developmental neuropsychiatry. New York: Guilford Press.

Ylvisaker, M. (1986). Language and communication disorders following pediatric head injury. Journal of Head Trauma Rehabilitation, 1, 48-56.

Ylvisaker, M. (1989). Cognitive and psychosocial outcome following head injury in children. In J.T. Hoff, T.E., Anderson, & T.M. Cole (Eds.), Mild to moderate head injury. London: Blackwell Scientific Publications, Inc.

Ylvisaker, M. (1995). Communication outcome in children and adolescents with traumatic brain injury. Neuropsychological Rehabilitation.

Frontal Lobe Injury in Children and Adults

Ackerly, S.S. (1964). A case of paranatal frontal lobe defect observed for thirty years. In J.M. Warren & K. Ackert (Eds.), The frontal granular cortex and behavior (pp. 192-218). New York: Mcgraw-Hill.

Anderson, S. W., Damasio, H., Tranel, D., & Damasio, A.R. (1988). Neuropsychological correlates of bilateral frontal lobe lesions in humans. Society for Neuroscience, 14, 1288-.

Bigler, E.D. (1988). Frontal lobe damage and neuropsychological assessment. Archives of Clinical Neuropsychology, 3, 279-297.

Eslinger, P.J., & Damasio, A.,R. (1985). Severe disturbance of higher cognition following bilateral frontal lobe oblation: Patient EVR. Neurology, 35, 1731-1741.

Eslinger, P.J., Grattan, L.M., Damasio, h>, & Damasio, A.R. (1992). Developmental consequences of childhood frontal lobe damage. Archives of Neurology, 49, 764-769.

Grattan, L.M., & Eslinger, P.J. (1991). Frontal lobe damage in children and adults: A comparative review. Developmental Neuropsychology, 7, 283-326.

Janowsky, J.S., Shimamura, A.P>, Kritchevsky, M. & Squire, L.R. (1989). Cognitive impairment following frontal lobe damage and its relevance to human amnesia. Behavioral Neuroscience, 103, 548-560.

Janowsky, J.S., Shimamura, A.P., & Squire (1989). Memory and metamemory: Comparisons between patients with frontal lobe lesions and amnesic patients. Psychobiology, 17, 3-11.

Mateer, C.A., & Williams, D. (1991). Effects of frontal lobe injury in childhood. Developmental Neuropsychology, 7, 359-376.

McGlynn, S.M., & Schacter, D.L. (1989). Unawareness of deficits in neuropsychological syndromes. Journal of Clinical and Experimental Neuropsychology, 11, 143-205.

Prigatano, G.P., & Schacter, D.L. (in press). Awareness of deficit after brain injury: Theoretical and clinical aspects. New York: Oxford University Press.

Schacter, D.L. (1990). Toward a cognitive neuropsychology of awareness: Implicit knowledge and anosagnosia. Journal of clinical and Experimental Neuropsychology, 12, 155-178.

Schacter, D.L., Glisky, E.L., & McGlynn, S.M. (1990). Impact of memory disorder on everyday life: Awareness of deficits and return to work. In D. Tupper & K. Cicerone (Eds.), The neuropsychology of everyday life< Vol. I, Theories and basic competencies. Boston: Martinus Nijhoff.

Schacter, D.L. (1987). Memory, amnesia, and frontal lobe dysfunction. Psychobiology, 15, 21-36.

Stuss, D.T., & Benson, D.F. (1986). The frontal lobes. New York: Raven Press.

Frontal Lobe Injury and Assessment
Functional Communication Assessment

Alexander, M.P., Benson, D.F., & Stuss, D.T. (1989). Frontal lobes and language. Brain and language, 37, 656-691.

Anderson, S.W., Damasio, H., Tranel, D., & Damasio, A.R. (1988). Neuropsychological correlates of bilateral frontal lobe lesions in humans. Society for Neuroscience, 14, 1288.

Anderson, S.W., & Tranel, D. (1989). Awareness of disease states following cerebral infarction, dementia, and head trauma: Standard assessment. The Clinical Neuropsychologist, 3, 327-339.

Baddeley, A.D., & Wilson, B. (1988). Frontal amnesia and the dysexecutive syndrome. Brain and Cognition, 7, 212-230.

Dennis, M. (1991). Frontal lobe function in childhood and adolescence: A heuristic for assessing attention regulation, executive control, and the intentional states important for social discourse. Developmental Neuropsychology, 7(3), 327-358.

Hartley, L.L. (1990). Assessment of functional communication. In D.E. Tupper & K.D. Cicerone (Eds.), The neuropsychology of everyday life: Assessment and basic competencies (pp. 125-168). Boston: Kluwer Academic Publishers.

Hartley, L.L.(1992). Assessment of functional communication. Seminars in Speech and Language, 13, 264-279.

Levin, H.S., Culhane, K.A., Hartman, J., Evankovich, K., Mattson, A.J., Harward, H., Ringolz, G., Ewing-Cobbs, L., & Fletcher, J.M. (1991). Developmental changes is performance on tests of purported frontal lobe functioning. Developmental Neuropsychology, 7, 377-395.

Lezak, M.D. (1982). The problem of assessing executive functions. International Journal of Psychology. 17, 281-197.

Lezak, M.D., (1983). Neuropsychological assessment. New York: Oxford University Press.

Lezak, M. (1987). Assessment for rehabilitation planning. In M. Meier, A.L. Benton, & L. Diller (Eds.), Neuropsychological rehabilitation (pp. 41-58). New York: Guilford Press.

Meichenbaum, D., Burland, S., & Gruson, L. (1985). Metacognitive assessment. In S. Yussen (Ed.), The Growth of Reflection in Children (pp. 3-30). Academic Press.

Stuss, D.T., & Buckle, L. (1992). Traumatic brain injury: Neuropsychological deficits and evaluation at different stages of recovery and in different pathologic subtypes. Journal of Head Trauma Rehabilitation, 7, 40-49.

Welsh, M.C., & Pennington, B.F. (1988). Assessing frontal lobe functioning in children: Views from developmental psychology. Developmental Neuropsychology, 4, 199-230.

Welsh, M.C., Pennington, B.F., & Groisser, D.B. (1991). A normative-developmental study of executive function: A window on prefrontal function in children. Developmental Neuropsychology, 7(2), 131-149.

Ylvisaker, M., Chorazy, A., Cohen, S., Nelson, J., Mastrelli, J., Molitor, C., Szekeres, S., & Valko, A (1990). Rehabilitative assessment following head injury in children. In M. Rosenthal, E. Griffith, M. Bond, & J.D. Miller (Eds.), Rehabilitation of the adult and child with traumatic brain injury. Philadelphia: FA Davis.

Ylvisaker, M., Hartwick, P., Ross, B., & Nussbaum, N. . Cognitive Assessment. In R. Savage & G. Wolcott (Eds.),(1993) Educational Dimensions of Acquired Brain Injury. Austin: Pro-Ed.

Organization and Memory

Baumeister, A., & Smith, S. (1979). Thematic elaboration and proximity in children's recall, organization, and long term retention of sectorial materials. Journal of Child Psychology, 28, 231-248.

Bjorklund, D. (1985). The role of conceptual knowledge in the development of organization in children's memory. In M. Pressley & C. Brainerd (Eds.), Basic processes in memory development (pp. 103-134). New York: Springer-Verlag.

Chi, M.T.H. (1978). Knowledge structures and memory development. In R. Siegler (Ed.), Children's thinking: What develops? (pp. 73-966). Hillsdale, N.J.: Lawrence Erlbaum. Assoc.

Lange, G. (1978). Organization-related processes in children's recall. In P. Ornstein (Ed.), Memory development in children (pp. 101-128). Hillsdale, NJ: Lawrence Erlbaum Assoc.

Levin, H.S., & Goldstein, F.C. (1986). Organization of verbal memory after severe head injury. Journal of Clinical and Experimental Neuropsychology, 8. 643-656.

Levin, H.S., Goldstein, F.C., High, W.M., & Williams, D. (1988). /automatic and effortful processing after severe closed head injury. Brain and Language, 7, 283-297.

Mandler, G. (1967). Organization and memory, In K,W. Spence & T. Spence (Eds.) The psychology of learning and motivation, Vol 1 Advances in research and theory (pp. 327-372), New York: Academic Press.

Moely, B. (1977). Organization of memory. In R. Kail & J. Hagen (Eds.), Perspectives on the development of memory and cognition (pp. 203-236). Hillsdale, NJ: Lawrence Erlbaum Assoc.

Moffat, N. (1984). Strategies of memory therapy. In B. Wilson & N. Moffat (Eds.), Clinical management of memory problems (pp. 63-88). Rockville, MD: Aspen System Corp.

Pressley, M., & Brainerd, C. (1985). Basic processes in memory development: Progress in cognitive development research. New York: Springer Verlag.

Schacter, D.L., & Glisky, E.L. (1986). Memory remediation: Restoration, alleviation, and the acquisition of domain-specific knowledge. In B. Uzzel & Y. Gross (Eds.), Clinical neuropsychology of intervention (pp. 257-282). Boston: Martinus Nijhoff.

Szekeres, S. (1988). Organization and recall in the young language impaired child. Doctoral Dissertation. University of Pittsburgh, Pittsburgh, PA.

Szekeres, S. (1992). Organization as an intervention target after traumatic brain injury, Seminars in Speech and Language, 13, 293-307.

Wilson, B., & Moffat, N. (Eds.) (1984). Clinical management of memory problems. Rockville, MD: Aspen Systems Corp.

Compensatory Strategies and Executive System Intervention
Alley, G.R., & Deshler, D.D. (1979). Teaching the learning disabled adolescent strategies and methods. Denver: Love Publishing Co.

Borkowski, J.G., Johnston, M.B., & Reid, M.K. (1986). Metacognition, motivation, and the transfer process, In S.J. Ceci (Ed.), Handbook of cognitive, social, and neuropsychological aspects of learning disabilities. Hillsdale, NJ: Lawrence Erlbaum, Assoc.

Brown, A.L. (1975). The development of memory: Knowing, knowing about knowing, and knowing how to know. In H.W. Reese (Ed)., Advances in child development and behavior. Vol. 10 (pp. 103-152). New York: Academic Press.

Flavell, J. (1985). Cognitive development, 2nd Edition. Englewood Cliffs, NJ: Prentice-Hall, Inc.

Forrest-Pressley, D.L., MacKinnon, G.E., & Waller, T.G. (Eds.) (1985). Metacognition, cognition, and human performance. Vol. 2. Instructional Practices. Orlando, Fla.: Academic Press.

Klonoff, P.S., O'Brien, K.P., Prigatano, G.P., Chiapello, D.A., & Cunningham, M. (1989). Cognitive retraining after traumatic brain injury and its role in facilitating awareness. Journal of Head Trauma Rehabilitation, 4(3), 37-45.

Meichenbaum, D. (1977). Cognitive behavior modification: An integrative approach. New York: Plenum Press.

Meichenbaum, D. (in press). The "potential" contributions of cognitive behavior modification to the rehabilitation of individuals with traumatic brain injury. Seminars in Speech and Language, 14.

Meichenbaum, D., & Asarnow, J. (1979). Cognitive-behavioral modification and metacognitive development:Implications for the classroom. In P.C. Kendall & S.D. Hollon (Eds.), Cognitive-behavioral interventions: Theory, research, and procedures (pp. 11-35). New York: Academic Press.

Pressley, M. (in press). Teaching cognitive strategies to brain-injured clients: The good information processing perspective. Seminars is Speech and Language, 14.

Pressley, M., & Associates (1990). Cognitive strategy instruction that really improves children's academic performance. Cambridge, MA: Brookline Books.

Pressley, M., Borkowski, J.G., & Schneider, W. (1989). Good information processing: What is it and what education can do to promote it. International Journal of Educational Research, 13, 857-867.

Pressley, M., & Levin, J.R. (Eds.) (1983a). Cognitive strategy training: Educational applications. New York: Springer Verlag.

Pressley, M., & Levin, J.R. (Eds.) (1983b). Cognitive strategy training: Psychological foundations. New York: Springer Verlag.

Ylvisaker, M., & Holland, A. (1985). Coaching, self-coaching, and the rehabilitation of head injury. In D. Johns (Ed.), Clinical management of neurogenic communicative disorders (pp. 243-257). Boston: Little-Brown.

Ylvisaker, M., Szekeres, S.F., & Hartwick, P. (1991). Cognitive rehabilitation following traumatic brain injury in children. In M. Tramontana & S. Hooper (Eds.), Advances in child neuropsychology, Vol. 1. New York: Springer Verlag.

Ylvisaker, M., Szekeres, S.F., Hartwick, P., & Tworek, P. (in press). Cognitive intervention. In R. Savage & G. Wolcott (Eds.),(1993) Educational Dimensions of Acquired Brain Injury. Austin: Pro-Ed.

Ylvisaker, M., Szekeres, S., Henry, K., Sullivan, D., & Wheeler, P. (1987). Topics in cognitive rehabilitation therapy. In M. Ylvisaker (Ed.), Community re-entry for head injured adults. Austin, TX: Pro-Ed.

Ylvisaker, M., & Szekeres, S. (1989). Metacognitive and executive impairments in head-injured children and adults. Topics in Language Disorders, 9(2), 34-49.

Social Skills Intervention

Bear, D. (1981). How to plan for generalization. Manhattan, KS: H&H Enterprises, Inc.

Braunling-McMorrow, d., Lloyd, K., & Fralish, K. (1986). Teaching social skills to head injured adults. Journal of Rehabilitation, 52, 39-44.

Brooks, D.N., & McKinlay, W. (1983). Personality and behavioral change after severe blunt head injury - a relative's view. Journal of Neurology, Neurosurgery, and Psychiatry, 46, 336-344.

Brotherton, F.A., Thomas, L.L., Wisotzek, I.E., & Milan, M.A. (1988). Social skills training in the rehabilitation of patients with traumatic closed head injury. Archives of Physical Medicine and Rehabilitation, 69, 827-832.

Carr, E.G., & Durand, V.M. (1985). The social-communicative basis of severe behavior problems in children. In S. Reiss & R. Bootzin (Eds.), Theoretical issues in behavior therapy (pp. 219-254). New York: Academic Press.

Collet-Klingenberg, L. & Chadsey-Rusch, J. (1991). Using a cognitive-process approach to teach social skills. Education and Training in Mental Retardation, 26, 258-270.

Foxx, R.M., Faw, G.D., & Webb, G. (1991). Producing generalization of adolescent's social skills with significant adults in a natural environment. Behavior Therapy, 22, 85-99.

Feeney, T.J., & Urbanczyk, B. (in press). Language as behavior or the myth of maladaptive behavior. In G. Wolcott & R.C. Savage (Eds.), Educational programming for children and young adults with acquired brain injury. Austin: Pro-Ed.

Gajar, A., Schloss, P.J., Schloss, C.N., & Thompson, C.K, (1984). Effects of feedback and self-monitoring on head trauma youths' conversation skills. Journal of Applied Behavior Analysis, 17, 3353-358.

Giles, G.M., Fussey, I., & Burgess, P. (1988). The behavioral treatment of verbal interaction skills following severe head injury: A single case study. Brain Injury, 2, 75-79.

Goldstein, A.P., Sprafkin, R.P., Gershaw, N.J., & Klein, P. (1980). Skillstreaming the adolescent: A structured learning approach to teaching prosocial skills. Champaign, IL: Research Press.

Gresham, F.M. (1988). Social skills: Conceptual and applied aspects of assessment, training, and social validation. In J.C. Witt, S.N. Elliot, & F.M. Gresham (Eds.), Handbook of behavior therapy in education. New York: Plenum Press.

Helffenstein, D., & Wechsler, R. (1982). The use of interpersonal process recall (IPR) in the remediation of interpersonal and communication skill deficits in the newly brain injured. Clinical Neuropsychology, 4, 139-143.

Lewis, F.D., Nelson, J., Nelson, C., & Reusink, P. (1988). Effects of three feedback contingencies on the socially inappropriate talk of a brain-injured adult, Behavior Therapy, 19, 203-211.

Malkmus D. (1988). Community reentry: Cognitive-communicative intervention in a social context. Topics in Language Disorders, 9(2), 50-66.

Marsh, N. V., & Knight, R. G. (1991). Behavioral assessment of social competence following severe head injury. Journal of Clinical and Experimental Neuropsychology, 13, 729-740.

McIntosh, S., Vaughn, S., & Zaragoza, N. (1991). A review of social interventions for students with learning disabilities. Journal of Learning Disabilities, 24, 451-458.

Schloss, P.J., Thompson, C.K., Gajar, A.H., & Schloss, C.N. (1985). Influence of self-monitoring on heterosexual conversational behaviors of head trauma youth. Applied Research in Mental Retardation, 6, 269-282.

Sheinker, J., & Sheinker, A. (1988). Metacognitive approach to social skills training. Rockville, MD: Aspen Publishers, Inc.

Stokes, T.F., & Osnes, P.G. (1986). Programming the generalization of children's social behavior. In P.S. Strain, M.J. Guralnick, & H.M. Walker (Eds.), Children's social behavior: Development, assessment, and modification. Academic Press, Inc.

Stokes, T.F., & Osnes, P.G. (1988). The developing applied technology of generalization and mainte-nance, In R.H. Horner, G. Dunlap, & R.L. Koegel (Eds.), Generalization and maintenance: Life-style changes in applied settings. Baltimore: Paul H. Brookes Publishing Co.

Waksman, S., Messmer, C.L., & Waksman, D.D. (1989). The Waksman Social Skills Curriculum: An assertive behavior program for adolescents. Austin, TX: Pro-Ed.

Walker, H.M., McConnell, S.M., Holmes, D., Todis, B., Walker, J., & Golden, N. (1988). The Walker Social Skills Curriculum: The ACCEPTS program. Austin, TX: Pro-Ed.

Walker, H.M., Todis, B., Holmes, D., & Horton, G. (1988). The Walker Social Skills Program: The ACCESS program: Adolescent curriculum for communication and effective social skills. Austin, TX: Pro-Ed.

Weddell, R., Oddy, M., & Jenkins, D. (1980). Social adjustment after rehabilitation: A two year follow-up of patients with severe head injury. Psychological Medicine, 10, 257-263.

Ylvisaker, M., Feeney, T., & Urbanczyk, B. (in press). Developing a positive communication culture for rehabilitation. In C.J. Durgin, J. Fryer, & N. Schmidt (Eds.), Brain injury rehabilitation: Clinical intervention and staff development techniques. Gaithersburg, MD: Aspen Publishers.

Ylvisaker, M., Szekeres, S., Haarbauer-Krupa, J., Urbanczyk, B., & Feeney, T. (in press). Speech and language intervention. In R. Savage and G. Wolcott (Eds.), (1994) Educational Dimensions of Acquired Brain Injury. Austin: Pro-Ed.

Ylvisaker, M., Urbanczyk, B., & Feeney, T. (1992). Social skills following traumatic brain injury. Seminars in Speech and Language, 13, 308-321.

Zaragoza, N., Vaughn, S., & McIntosh, R. (1991). Social skills interventions and children with behavior problems: A review. Behavioral Disorders, 16, 260-275.

School Re-Entry

Blosser, J.L., & DePompei, R. (1989). The head injured student returns to school: Recognizing and treating deficits. Topics in Language Disorders, 9, 67-77.

Cohen, S.B. (1986). Educational reintegration and programming for children with head injuries. Journal of Head Trauma Rehabilitation, 1, 22-29.

DePompei, R., & Blosser, J.L. (1986). Strategies for helping head-injured children successfully return to school. Language, Speech, and Hearing Services in the Schools, 18, 292-300.

Hall, D.E., & DePompei, R. (1986). Implications for head injured re-entering higher education. Cognitive Rehabilitation, 4, 6-8.

Mira, M., Tyler, J., & Tucker, B. (1988). Traumatic head injury in children: A guide for schools. Kansas City, KA: University of Kansas Medical Center.

Rosen, C.D., & Gerring, J.P. (1992). Head trauma: Educational reintegration (second edition). San Diego: Singular Press.

Savage, R.C. (1987). Educational issues for the head-injured adolescent and young adult. Journal of Head Trauma Rehabilitation, 2, 1-10.

Savage, R.C., & Carter, R.R. (1991). Family and return to school. In J.M. Williams & T. Kay (Eds.), Head injury: A family matter. Baltimore: Paul H. Brookes Publishing Co.

Savage, R.C. & Wolcott, G.F. (Eds.) (1994) Educational Dimensions of Acquired Brain Injury. Austin: Pro-Ed.

Savage, R.C. & Wolcott, G.F. (Eds.) (1988). An educator's manual: What educators need to know about students with traumatic brain injury. (Second Edition). Southborough, MA: NHIF.

Telzrow, C.F. (1987). Management of academic and educational problems in head injury. Journal of Learning Disabilities, 20, 536-545.

Tyler, J.S. (1995). Serving students with traumatic brain injuries in the learning disabilities classroom. LD Forum.

Tyler, J.S., & Mira, M.P. (in press). Educational modifications for students with head injuries. Teaching Exceptional Children.

Ylvisaker, M., Hartwick, P., & Stevens, M.B. (1991). School reentry following head injury: Managing the transition from hospital to school. Journal of Head Trauma Rehabilitation, 6, 10-22.

Cognitive-Language Assessment

Baxter, R., Cohen, S., & Ylvisaker, M. (1985). Comprehensive cognitive assessment. In M. Ylvisaker (Ed.), Head injury rehabilitation: Children and adolescents (pp. 247-274). San Diego: College-Hill Press.

Buschke, H., & Fuld, P.A. (1974). Evaluating storage, retention, and retrieval in disordered memory and learning. Neurology, 1019-1025.

Denckla, M.B., & Rudel, R. (1976). Rapid "automatized" naming (R.A.N.): Dyslexia differentiated from other learning disabilities. Neuropsychologia, 14, 471-479.

DiSimoni, F. (1978). The Token Test for Children. Allen, TX: DLM-Teaching Resources.

Dunn, L., & Dunn, L. (1981). Peabody Picture Vocabulary Test-Revised. Minneapolis, MN: American Guidance Service.

Gaddes, W.H., & Crocket, D.J. (1975). The Spreen-Benton Aphasia Tests: Normative data as a measure of normal language development. Brain and Language, 2, 257-280.

Gardner, M.F. (1979). Expressive One-Word Picture Vocabulary Test. Novato, CA: Academic Therapy Publications.

Goodglass, H., & Kaplan, E. (1972). Boston Diagnostic Aphasia Examination. Philadelphia: Lea & Febiger.

Hammill, D. (1985). Detroit Tests of Learning Aptitude (DTLA-2). Austin, TX: Pro-Ed.

Jorgenson, C., Barrett, M., Huisingh, R., & Zachman, L. (1981). The Word Tests. Moline, IL: Lingui Systems.

Prutting, C.A., & Kirchner, D.M. (1987). A clinical appraisal of the pragmatic aspects of language. Journal of Speech and Hearing Disorders, 52, 105-109.

Ross, J.D., & Ross, C.M. (1976). Ross Test of Higher Cognitive Processes. Novata, CA: Academic Therapy Publications.

Semel, E., Wiig, E.H., & Secord, W. (1987). Clinical Evaluation of Language Fundamentals-Revised. San Antonio, TX: The Psychological Corporation.

Wechsler, D. (1987). Wechsler Memory Scale - Revised. New York: Psychological Corporation.

Wiig, E.H., & Secord, W. (1988). Test of Language Competence-Expanded Edition. San Antonio, TX: The Psychological Corporation.

Woodcock, R., & Johnson, M. (1989). Woodcock - Johnson Psycho-Educational Test Battery. Allen Park, TX: DLM Teaching Resources.